MANUAL
OF
NUCLEAR MEDICINE IMAGING

MANUAL
OF
NUCLEAR MEDICINE IMAGING

Christopher C. Kuni
René P. duCret

1997
Thieme
New York • Stuttgart

Thieme Medical Publishers, Inc.
381 Park Avenue South
New York, NY 10016

MANUAL OF NUCLEAR MEDICINE IMAGING
René P. duCret, M.D.
Christopher C. Kuni, M.D.

Library of Congress Cataloging-in-Publication Data on file

Printed in the United States of America

5 4 3 2 1

TMP ISBN 0-86577-568-0
GTV ISBN 3-13-103741-5

To Suzy, Bill, Alexandra, Nora, Kitty, and Curious.
— CCK

To Susan J. Roe, M.D.
— RdC

Preface

The purpose of this book is to provide a concise, readable, and portable text for residents, fellows, and those in the general practice of radiology. Those outside the field of radiology should also benefit from this manual, since the text is focused on the most clinically relevant material. Unlike other short reviews of the subject, this book contains a large number of images from current clinical practice creating a unique resource for quick and easy reference. The book is organized by organ systems and also includes information on quality control requirements, dosimetry, physiology of tracers, physics, instrumentation, and radiochemistry. Appendices present guidelines for procedures, lists of radiopharmaceuticals and isotopes used in scintigraphy, and rules and regulations from the Nuclear Regulatory Commission. Throughout the work we focus upon state of the art procedures and minimize discussion of tests which have fallen into disfavor or disuse. The end of each chapter contains a list of suggested reading which includes up-to-date references, comprehensive reviews and some classic reading in the field.

Nuclear medicine continues to thrive due to the utility of a number of established protocols and the development of new cost-efficient procedures. The most promising developments are discussed and key references are represented. For instance, cardiac imaging is benefiting from the development of thallium re-injection and dual isotope techniques. We also have an FDA approved antibody for oncologic imaging and are using sestamibi for breast imaging and fluorodeoxglucose imaging for a variety of tumors. In addition, high-energy collimators have been developed for FDG SPECT imaging, detection of infection has benefited from HMPAO white cell labeling and the development of new kits has allowed rapid diagnosis and no exposure to blood products. Patients at high risk for renovascular hypertension continue to benefit from more concise protocols for angiotensin converting enzyme inhibitor studies. Stronium-89 has been approved for use of palliation of bone pain. In-111 pentetreotide is now used routinely for imaging neuroendocrine tumors and is beginning to supplant the use of I-131 MIBG.

This affordable and concise pocket book is meant to be read cover to cover. The book stresses procedures that are doing well in nuclear medicine and the best of the new developments. We hope that readers will enjoy seeing images from clinical practice that complement the concise text and find this a practical quick resource in the routine practice of nuclear medicine.

Acknowledgments

William H. Thompson, M.D., chairman of the radiology department at the University of Minnesota, was enthusiastic and encouraging during all phases of this project; we deeply appreciate his support. Robert J. Boudreau, M.D., Ph.D., provided clinical and administrative input as head of the nuclear medicine service. Charla Zaccardi, with assistance from Clemmer Wait, expertly created the text and tables from our dictations and sketches. Walter Gutzmer and Rhonda Dragan produced the photographs and drawings. Many technologists, including James Tennison, CNMT, chief nuclear medicine technologist at the University of Minnesota Academic Health Center, contributed clinical images.

Contents

Chapter 1

Introduction

There is a fundamental difference between the physiological approach of nuclear medicine and the anatomic approach of transmission imaging for the diagnosis and treatment of disease. Many subspecialties of medicine today have roots in anatomical or static approaches to disease. The use of such an ontological approach to disease suggests that the disease process is an entity that can be demonstrated by gross pathology or histopathology. Foundations for this approach lie in the nineteenth century work of Virchow, who described cellular abnormalities as the basis for disease processes. Today, the contributions of biochemistry and physiology play a complementary role to anatomy in diagnosis and treatment. Using this approach the clinician observes and measures functional abnormalities and describes disease in terms of abnormal biochemical or physiological function. Since nuclear medicine has played a role in moving from the anatomic to the molecular level of diagnosis, the term molecular nuclear medicine has been suggested. It is of interest to review the historical events that built the foundation of the modern clinical nuclear medicine practice.

Within a year of Wilhelm Roentgen's discovery of x-rays, Henri Becquerel looked for an alternative to the Crookes cathode ray tube for production of x-rays. He showed that uranium salts which were exposed to sunlight darkened photographic plates. However, when these uranium salts were not exposed to sunlight and were placed in a dark drawer with photographic plates the same result was observed. Marie Curie investigated this new type of penetrating radiation further. In 1898, 1 year after Thomson's discovery of the electron, Curie discovered two elements in uranium ore pitchblende that she named Polonium and Radium. The unit of radioactivity produced by a gram of radium was subsequently named a curie. The first use of radium for radiation therapy was in 1901, and in 1905 radium was placed into a thyroid goiter for treatment.

In 1911 the Hungarian George de Hevesy used lead-212 and a gold leaf electroscope to demonstrate that left over food was

1

being recycled into his meals in a boarding house in which he resided. It is de Hevesy who is now regarded as the inventor of the tracer principle and as the "father of nuclear medicine." He used the artificial isotope P-32 and a counter developed by Geiger in 1928 to study tracer metabolism in animals and later in humans. In 1924 Blumgart and Weiss measured the "velocity of circulation" by intravenous injection of Bi-214 in humans. Shortly thereafter in 1931 Ernest Lawrence invented the cyclotron, and in 1934 Marie Curie and Frederick Joliot suggested that isotopes could be produced by bombardment of appropriate elements with protons, neutrons, and deuterons. In 1937 P-32 was used to treat leukemia and I-128 was used to study thyroid physiology. Carbon-14 became available for biomedical research after World War II. Enrico Fermi and colleagues produced a number of radioactive isotopes through their work in the Manhattan Project.

The time after World War II was the beginning of what some have called the modern era of nuclear medicine. A number of developments took place that allowed the use of these new radioactive isotopes for imaging in human subjects. Benedict Cassen developed the rectilinear scanner in the late 1950s using a thick sodium iodide crystal linked to a mechanical system which recorded activity by either a pen moving over paper or a light moving over film. This slow and limited resolution method did not allow dynamic imaging of a tracer. This drawback was solved by Hal Anger using a relatively large sodium iodide crystal contaminated with a small amount of thallium to allow scintillations at room temperature. The development of the Mo-99/Tc-99m generator in 1965 provided a ready source of a gamma emitter which was suitable to imaging with the Anger camera. In the late 1960s the concept of single photon emission computed tomography (SPECT) was developed by Kuhl and Edwards. The early work on the reconstruction of SPECT images significantly preceded the work of Hounsfield in 1973. The clinical use of computed tomography would in turn later enhance SPECT imaging. Imaging with positron emitting radionuclides was suggested in 1951 by Wrenn and laid the foundation for PET imaging.

The development of the proper radiopharmaceutical for use with the new Anger scintillation camera played a major role in developing the modern practice of nuclear medicine. The term *radiopharmaceutical* refers to an FDA-approved combination of a radionuclide and a ligand that determines the biodistribution within the body. Two years after the discovery of technetium by Perrier and Segre in 1937, Tc-99m was discovered. Tc-99m has become the most commonly used isotope for emission imaging. Tc-99m is a short-lived nuclear isomer with a half life of 6.03 hours and is available from uranium fission. It primarily emits gamma photons, but occasionally has a betalike effect on tissue by emitting low-energy Auger electrons. Since its energy of emission is 140 keV it is well suited to imaging with the 3/8-inch-thick sodium iodide crystal which is commonly used today.

The first intravenous use of sodium pertechnetate in a human subject was made in 1961. Two developments that then simplified the use of pertechnetate were a generator system that could be eluted with saline and single vial kits that contained stannous ion reducing agent. Since technetium is a transition metal with a complex chemical behavior, and since technetium can assume any oxidation state from 0 to +7, the development of new technetium radiopharmaceuticals remains a significant challenge. Nevertheless nearly 90% of diagnostic nuclear medicine procedures today use Tc-99m radiopharmaceuticals.

Some landmarks in the development of the use of Tc-99m were the development of sulfur colloid in 1964, the production of aerosols in 1965, the use of macroaggregated albumin in 1966, and the development of DTPA kits in 1970. Developments in the 1970s included the use of labeled albumin, red blood cells, DMSA, MDP, and IDA derivatives. More recent developments in the 1980s and 1990s were the development of sestamibi, MAG3, teboroxime, tetrofosmin and ECD. The development of these various ligands for Tc-99m continues to expand a medical specialty that is based on the measurement of in vivo regional chemistry in the human body. The descriptive title "molecular nuclear medicine," a term suggested by Henry Wagner, does indeed seem appropriate for the modern era of nuclear medicine.

There are a number of regulations and suggestions that now guide the dispensing of radiopharmaceuticals, and these regulations are enforced by the FDA and the NRC, as well as by local and state regulatory bodies. The dosage must be ordered by an authorized user and copies of the test requisition and the dosage must be kept. All quality control procedures must be carried out and documented and the patient dose must then be assayed in a dose calibrator. The dose that is administered should be within 10% of the dose that was ordered. Misadministrations may involve use of the wrong radiopharmaceutical or wrong method of administration or the wrong patient. The guidelines for handling and reporting misadministrations are covered in the Code of Federal Regulations and are more complex when the doses involve a therapeutic administration or a diagnostic dose involving iodine. Adverse reactions to radiopharmaceutical products are extremely uncommon and usually mild. Allergic reactions due to the development of human antimouse antibody responses to radiolabeled antibodies remain a concern. The overall rarity of adverse reactions in nuclear medicine was recently reported by a study that reviewed the total number of adverse reactions to 773,525 administrations of radiopharmaceuticals. The prevalence of adverse reactions was approximately two per 100,000 administrations. For nonradioactive drugs such as dipyridamole and glucagon the number of adverse reactions was slightly higher.

A more common concern regarding radiopharmaceutical products is the question regarding pregnancy or breast-feeding. A dose to the fetus or to a child should always be kept as low as reasonably achievable, but nuclear medicine diagnostic procedures may be performed during pregnancy. Radioiodine administration should be avoided especially after the tenth week of gestation due to the ability of the fetal thyroid gland to concentrate radioiodine at this point. Breast-feeding should be discontinued permanently or for a minimum of 3 weeks following administration of I -131, Ga-67, or Tl-201. In general, breast-feeding should also be discontinued for at least 12 hours following administration of Tc-99m-labeled radiopharmaceuticals.

Another common problem is the calculation of dosages for the pediatric population. Although body weight can be used as a guide, body surface area would be most accurate for determining pediatric dosage. Since this formulation is impractical, a number of formulae based on age have been suggested. Unfortunately, some of these formulae may overestimate dose in the neonatal period. A simplified formula that is widely used and provides suitable image quality involves giving patients who are up to 5 years old one quarter of the adult dose and giving patients who are 5–10 years old one half the adult dose. Patients who are 10–15 years of age can be given three quarters of an adult dose and those 15 years or older may receive an adult dose.

Before the application of radiopharmaceuticals is discussed in relation to various organ systems, a word should be said about the way that these studies play a role in the diagnostic process. The general method of evaluating the benefit of a diagnostic test in terms of sensitivity and specificity is well known. Sensitivity is simply the proportion of positive tests in patients who have the disease and specificity is the proportion of negative tests in those patients who do not have the disease. The term *accuracy* is also frequently utilized and reflects the proportion of correct test outcomes (true positives and true negatives) relative to all test outcomes. These terms, however, do not adequately describe whether a test adds significant information to the diagnostic process. Of greater interest is the predictive value of a positive or negative test, and this can be calculated using Bayes' theorem. Bayes' theorem relates the pretest probability of disease to the posttest or posterior probability of disease. Thus, a test with a certain sensitivity and specificity will produce various posttest probabilities of disease given the prevalence of that disease in the population that was studied. Bayes' theorem can be thought of as inverse probability since it gives the proportion of patients who are likely to have a given disease relative to the test results. Bayes' theorem has been applied to diagnostic studies in clinical medicine since 1959. The use of this theorem underscores the importance of viewing results in the context of the population to which a test has been applied and describes the diagnostic process as propabilistic. The information content of a diagnostic nuclear medicine procedure provides the clinician with an increase or decrease of a certainty that a given patient does or does not have a disease. In general, in order to provide a significant amount of diagnostic information, a diagnostic test must have a relatively higher accuracy when applied to a population with a low prevalence of disease.

The evaluation of diagnostic testing has an impact on the cost of nuclear medicine procedures. Today the cost of diagnostic or therapeutic procedures may seem loosely related to the price which is billed. The amount paid by insurers may be only a fraction of the amount billed by providers. Furthermore, costs vary greatly from facility to facility and depend on available resources. Today, indirect medical costs (e.g., the costs to society) play a significant role in an environment that includes managed care. In the following chapters we attempt to emphasize the description of those nuclear medicine procedures that are widely available and generally considered to be cost-effective in the delivery of medical care.

References

Chapman EM. History of the discovery and early use of radioactive iodine. *JAMA* 1983; 250:2042–2044.

Diamond GA, Forrester JS. Analysis of probability as an aid in the clinical diagnosis of coronary artery disease. *N Engl J Med* 1979; 300:1350.

Eckelman WC, Richards P. Instant[99m]Tc compounds. *Nucl Med* 1971; 10:245–251.

Graham LS, Kereiakes JG, Harris C, Cohen MB. Nuclear medicine from Becquerel to the present. *Radiographics* 1989; 9:1189–1202.

Griner PF, Mayewski RJ, Mushlin AI, Greenland P. Selection and interpretation of diagnostic tests and procedures. *Ann Intern Med* 1981; 94:557–592.

Hounsfield GN. Computerized transverse axial scanning (tomography): I. Description of system. *Br J Radiol* 1973; 46:1016–1022.

Jaszczak RJ, Huard D, Murphy P, Burdine J. Radionuclide emission computed tomography with a scintillation camera. *J Nucl Med* 1976; 17:551.

Kuhl DE, Edwards RQ. Image separation radioisotope scanning. *Radiology* 1963; 80:653–662, .

McNeil BJ, Keeler E, Adelstein SJ. Primer on certain elements of medical decision making. *N Engl J Med* 1975;293:211–215.

McNeil BJ. Socioeconomic forces affecting medicine: times of increased retrenchment and accountability. *Semin Nucl Med* 1993; 23:3–8.

Ransohoff DF, Freinstein AR. Problems of spectrum and bias in evaluating the efficacy of diagnostic tests. *N Engl J Med* 1978; 299:926–930.

Roentgen WK. On a new kind of rays (trans). *Nature* 1896; 53:274–276.

Richards P, Tucker WD, Srivastava SC. Introduction: technetium-99m: an historical perspective. *Int J Appl Rad Isot* 1982; 33(10):793–799.

Serge E, Seaborg GT. Discovery of technetium. *Phys Rev* 1938:54.

Siddiqui AR. *Nuclear Imaging in Pediatrics.* Year Book Medical Publishers, Chicago, 1985, pp. 1–6.

Wagner HN Jr. Present and future applications of radiopharmaceuticals from generator-produced radioisotopes. *Int Atomic Energy Agency* 1971:163.

Chapter 2

Cardiovascular System

Two procedures now predominate in the scintigraphic evaluation of cardiac function: evaluation of myocardial perfusion and gated blood pool imaging. Infarct avid imaging with Tc99m-pyrophosphate is less frequently done but will also be discussed.

Myocardial Perfusion

Thallium-201 is a cyclotron-produced radionuclide with biokinetic properties similar to potassium. Uptake in the myocardium is by the sodium-potassium ATPase system. The affinity of this system for ionic thallium is actually higher than for rubidium or potassium. Extraction of thallium from the blood is nearly 90%, with each pass through the coronary bed resulting in accumulation of approximately 3.5% of the injected dose within the myocardium at rest. Approximately 4.4% of the injected dose localizes within the heart after treadmill testing. Infusion of dipyridamole causes even greater accumulation of injected thallium within the heart by a factor of at least 1.3, but it also produces greater splanchnic accumulation of activity.

Thallium-201 decays by electron capture and the majority of photons produced are from the daughter product, mercury-201, which produces x-rays in the range of 68 to 83 kev. If multiple channels are available, the thallium gamma emission at 135 and 167 kev can be included to increase overall count rates by 10 to 15%. A typical setup using a gamma camera with a 3/8-inch crystal would include a 20% window on the mercury x-rays and a 20% window on the 167-kev thallium gamma. The administered dose is limited by the radiation burden to the critical organ, which in the case of thallium is the kidney. With injection of 3 mCi of thallium-201 at rest or 4 mCi at exercise, the radiation burden to the kidneys has been estimated at 3–5 rad. Although the renal medulla receives the highest dose following a thallium injection, significant doses also result to the lens and the gonads. Although the kidneys are the critical organ, less than

10% of injected thallium is excreted through the urinary tract within 24 hours, resulting in a relatively long effective half-life in the body of approximately 56 hours.

The phenomenon of thallium redistribution is central to the understanding of image interpretation. Within 10 minutes of the thallium injection a small reservoir of less than 1% of the injected dose remains within the blood. This reservoir is in equilibrium with the myocardium. Uptake into the myocardium initially is dependent on perfusion and cellular extraction, and following a rapid rise to peak activity within the myocardium there is a prolonged period of myocardial washout of thallium that reflects myocardial viability. This washout is slower in zones of decreased myocardial viability due to hypoperfusion. Ischemic myocardium will thus show lower initial concentration of thallium but also a lesser degree of washout. Normal myocardium will show more intense homogeneous thallium uptake with a higher washout rate. Because of the higher washout rate the normal myocardium may show thallium intensity on delayed images that is similar to that of ischemic myocardium. This interval change between initial difference and subsequent equilibration of thallium activity in the myocardium is generally termed *redistribution.* Areas of scarring have low initial perfusion and therefore low initial levels of thallium activity, but they also show washout that is comparable to the rates of loss of thallium activity from normal myocardium. Thus myocardial zones that include areas of fibrosis would demonstrate fixed photopenic defects and show no redistribution (Fig. 2-1). Eating between exercise and rest studies should be discouraged since insulin release causes the NaK ATPase transport system to drive potassium intracellularly, causing increased washout of thallium. This increased washout rate can cause ischemic myocardium to appear as a relatively fixed defect. The differentiation of fixed from reversible defects can be enhanced by either a delayed acquisition of images at rest or reinjection of thallium prior to the resting study. Occasionally, severely ischemic myocardium will show very low initial thallium activity and persistently low activity by the 3- or 4-hour rest acquisition point. These areas will appear fixed at 4 hours but may reach the intensity of normal myocardium by 24 hours, thus showing redistribution and viability. The disadvantage of the 24 hour acquisition is not only the acquisition of three sets of images over a prolonged period but also the decreased count rates seen at 24 hours. **Reinjection** of thallium prior to rest image acquisition is more feasible and is an effective means of differentiating viable myocardium from scar. Two mCi of thallium are typically given during exercise and 1 mCi is given prior to rest acquisition. Improved image quality at a slightly higher dose to the patient can be obtained with 3 mCi at exercise and 2 mCi prior to a rest image acquisition (Fig. 2-2). **Reinjection** of thallium allows for a more accurate representation of perfusion and cellular uptake during the resting period with significantly increased image quality of the resting image. Up to 50% of apparent fixed lesions may show redistribution following reinjection of thallium.

Although reinjection enhances the detection of ischemic myocardium, not all patients with ischemia will show redistribu-

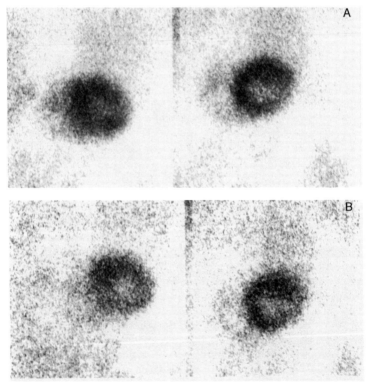

Figure 2-1. *continued*

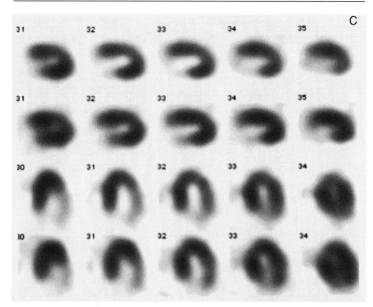

Figure 2-1. Planar stress (A), rest (B), and SPECT (C) thallium-201 imaging following treadmill exercise. The anterior planar images are relatively unremarkable. The LAO 45-degree images reveal a persistent abnormality of the posterolateral myocardium. SPECT images in the sagittal and horizontal long axis reveal a fixed posterior abnormality and also show mild redistribution involving the anterior, apical, and lateral myocardium.

tion by the reinjection study. Persistent perfusion or metabolic abnormalities in myocardium may account for apparently fixed defects even with the reinjection technique. Delayed thallium imaging at 24 hours or longer after the stress phase has been proposed as a means to deal with this phenomenon. Although detection of ischemia may be slightly enhanced, there is marked image degradation because of low count rates and poor object-to-background ratios at markedly delayed imaging times. In addition, not all abnormalities on a thallium myocardial scan are secondary to epicardial coronary artery disease. Abnormalities on stress and rest images have been documented in patients with **congestive or hypertrophic cardiomyopathy, Chagas disease, sarcoidosis, aortic stenosis, coronary vasospasm,** and **infiltrative** and **metastatic disease. Left bundle branch block** is well

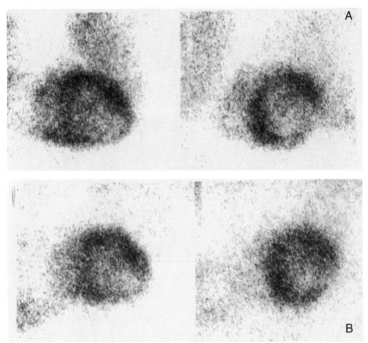

Figure 2-2. *continued*

documented as a cause of septal redistribution in the absence of large-vessel coronary disease.

Proper interpretation of thallium myocardial studies demands an understanding of a variety of **artifacts** that can be detected on planar and tomographic imaging. Apical thinning and decreased activity in the posterior portion of the septum and inferior wall are frequently seen. The infradiaphragmatic structures can attenuate the inferior wall. Visceral activity may occasionally be significant (Fig. 2-3) and increase the apparent counts in the inferior wall during a SPECT (single photon emission) acquisition. Because mercury x-rays have a relatively poor ability to penetrate soft-tissue, there can be marked attenuation by overlying soft-tissue structures such as the breast (Fig. 2-4). In general, some image degradation can be expected in obese patients because of relatively impaired flux of mercury x-rays (Fig. 2-5). Increased thallium deposition in skeletal muscle or in the papil-

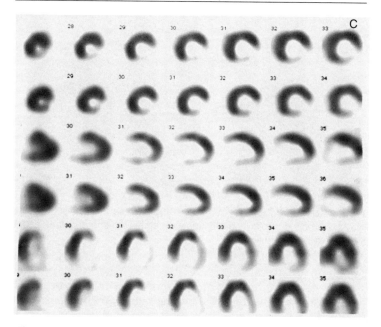

Figure 2-2. Exercise planar and SPECT thallium-201 imaging with reinjection. Anterior and LAO 45-degree images following 3 mCi of intravenous thallium-201 (A) show increased lung uptake and a dilated left ventricle. Perfusion abnormalities are present in the inferoapical and posterolateral myocardium. Increased lung uptake is a sign of global left ventricular dysfunction. Planar images obtained after reinjection with 2 mCi of thallium-201 (B) show resolution of lung uptake. SPECT images (C) show a relatively fixed abnormality of the lateral myocardium with evidence of redistribution involving the inferior and, to a lesser degree, anterior myocardium.

lary muscles is occasionally confusing. In addition, craniocaudal movement of the heart during a SPECT acquisition can cause significant image degradation. Inconsistent identification of the long axis of the heart prior to image reconstruction can also cause spurious abnormalities when comparison is made between the stress and rest images (Fig. 2-6). Implantable hardware such as automatic defibrillator devices must also be taken into consideration. Artifacts may also be caused by inconsistent application of cutoff frequencies for reconstruction filters (Fig. 2-7).

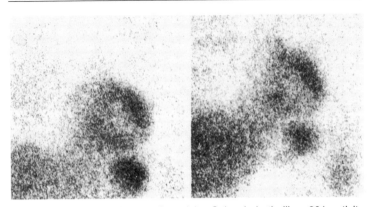

Figure 2-3. Infradiaphragmatic activity. Splanchnic thallium-201 activity may be prominent following dipyridamole administration and may affect interpretation of the inferior wall.

Patients who are about to undergo thallium myocardial scintigraphy should fast for at least 6 hours when possible. Intake of food should also be discouraged between the stress and rest images because insulin release causes potassium to be driven into the cells, enhancing washout of intracellular thallium. Reduced splanchnic blood flow is desirable at all times because infradiaphragmatic activity can degrade image acquisition.

The goal of exercise should be to raise the patient's myocardial oxygen demand. Whenever possible this is achieved by use of the Bruce protocol on an exercise treadmill. This aggressive protocol involves increase of both speed and incline of the treadmill in 3-minute stages. Use of a bicycle ergometer when necessary may result in less than optimal exercise levels. The product of peak heart rate and peak systolic pressure ("double product") gives an indication of the level of exercise achieved. Ideally, a double product of 24,000 or greater should be achieved. Thallium injection is made through a heparin lock 1 minute before termination of exercise. Eighty-five percent of maximum predicted heart rate should ideally be reached. Clinical symptoms or EKG changes may terminate exercise. Image acquisition should begin within 5 to 10 minutes of peak stress. Images should be recorded in the anterior, 45 degrees left anterior oblique and 70 degrees left anterior oblique view. Images are generally obtained

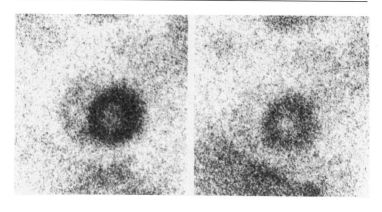

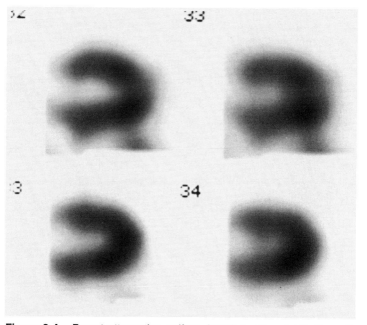

Figure 2-4. Breast attenuation artifact. Anterior wall redistribution with normal coronary angiography. Breast tissue can often be identified as an overlying curvilinear photopenic defect on planar images.

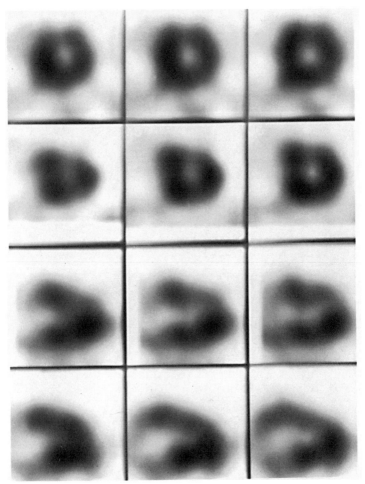

Figure 2-5. Obesity artifact. Female patient, 5 ft, 3 in, 221 lbs, and with normal ECG and angiogram. Multiple artifactual defects are present with and without redistribution (stress images above rest images).

in the supine position although various oblique and lateral decubitus views have been suggested as a means of decreasing infradiaphragmatic attenuation and breast attenuation of the myocardial activity. Planar images are obtained for a total of

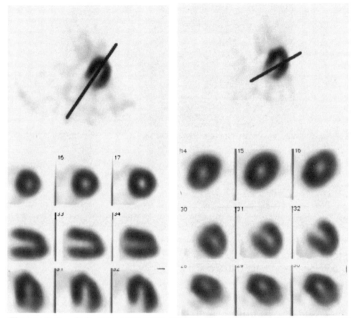

Figure 2-6. Axis reconstruction artifact. The long axis for reconstruction of SPECT short axis, sagittal long axis, and horizontal long axis images must be carefully selected. SPECT images here are normal following proper axis selection, but become markedly distorted with lateral deviation of the axis.

between 200,000 and 400,000 counts for a total acquisition time of 8 to 10 minutes per view. SPECT acquisition is then made with a gamma camera revolving in a 180-degree arch from the patient's RAO to the LPO position. Acquisition can be either in continuous or step-wise (e.g., every 6 degrees) modes. Delayed images are obtained in a similar manner after reinjection of 1 to 2 mCi of thallium. Reinjection can be made either after the stress image acquisition is completed or immediately prior to the rest image acquisition. Both planar and SPECT images are then recorded after careful attention is made to finding the longitudinal axis of the left ventricle for tomographic reconstruction. The anterior planar image can be used to assess lung uptake by comparing activity in the left lung with anterolateral wall activity. A

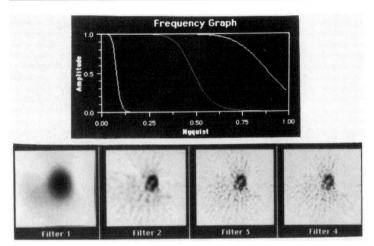

Figure 2-7. Artifacts may be due to filters used in reconstruction. Here cutoff frequencies of 0.1, 0.5, 0.9, and no filter were used. Excessive smoothing is apparent with a cutoff frequency of 0.1.

lung-to-heart ratio of greater than 0.5 is abnormal at heart rates greater than 140 beats per minute (Fig. 2-8). Abnormal lung-heart ratios may be seen with low heart rates. In the setting of adequate myocardial oxygen demand increased lung uptake signifies global left ventricular dysfunction during exercise and is a poor prognostic indicator.

Planar images are also useful for assessing abnormal soft-tissue attenuation or areas of increased infradiaphragmatic activity. Infradiaphragmatic activity is especially prominent with use of intravenous dipyridamole infusion or stress imaging. **Dipyridamole** is an adenosine deaminase inhibitor. **Adenosine** is a potent vasodilator of the resistance vessels in the coronary bed. The effect is usually obtained by infusing 0.14 mg/kg of dipyridamole per minute for a total of 4 minutes while monitoring the patient for EKG changes and a drop in blood pressure. The increase in coronary blood flow is 3 to 5 times more than the normal levels, resulting in myocardial uptake of approximately 8 to 10% of the injected dose. Preparations containing **xanthines** such as **theophylline** or caffeine should be withheld for at least 24 hours prior to dipyridamole infusion. Xanthines block the adenosine receptor sites. Intravenous administration of

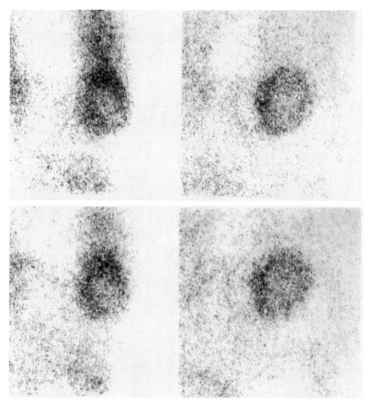

Figure 2-8. Abnormal lung-to-heart activity ratio. Increased lung uptake with a lung-to-heart ratio of greater than 0.5 is seen in this exercise thallium-201 image (above). A lung-to-heart ratio of greater than 0.5 is considered abnormal at heart rates faster than 140 bpm. Partial resolution of increased lung uptake is seen on the planar rest image in this patient.

aminophylline (usually a 250 mg bolus followed by 250mg drip) is effective in rapidly reversing any undesirable side effects caused by dipyridamole infusion. Thallium is injected within 4 minutes of the termination of dipyridamole infusion, and imaging is begun within 5 to 10 minutes (Fig. 2-9). Adenosine is an alternative to dipyridamole infusion because of its short half-life, but patients must be more carefully monitored for side effects.

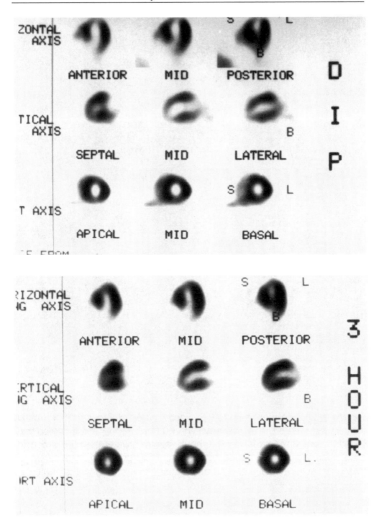

Figure 2-9. Dipyridamole thallium imaging with reinjection. Selected SPECT images are presented from the horizontal, sagittal, and short-axis reconstructions. The patient received 3 mCi of thallium-201 following dipyridamole infusion and was reinjected with 2 mCi of thallium-201 prior to rest imaging. There is evidence of moderate apical thallium redistribution. Note the presence of infradiaphragmatic activity following dipyridamole infusion.

Both quantitative methods and computer display options optimize the interpretation of the stress and rest images. Since planar images are obtained for a set number of counts, only relative changes in myocardial intensity should be noted. Tomographic images are standardized for maximum pixel intensity and may therefore be more directly compared for both homogeneity and intensity of thallium distribution. Quantitative techniques such as bull's-eye display can be helpful but should not be used without evaluation of planar or tomographic images. Computer display of stress and rest images provides helpful color gradients and variable background subtraction to enhance detection of differences in thallium intensity. A cine display of the acquisition phase is also helpful to show any craniocaudal movement of the heart during SPECT imaging.

Thallium imaging provides useful information not only for diagnosis of coronary artery disease but also for prognosis in patients with suspected disease and those who are posttherapy. Overall the sensitivity of the electrocardiogram is approximately 60%, with a specificity of approximately 80%. Electrocardiography is relatively insensitive in detection of posterior and inferior myocardial disease and loses specificity when ST changes occur in patients who have left ventricular hypertrophy or who are receiving digitalis. The sensitivity of exercise thallium imaging using either qualitative or quantitative techniques ranges from approximately 70% for single-vessel disease to 95% for three-vessel disease, with an average of approximately 85%. Specificity is impaired by the types of artifacts discussed earlier but also is in the range of 85%. Overall sensitivity is greatest for disease involving the left anterior descending coronary artery and lowest for circumflex disease where sensitivity approaches approximately 50%. There are theoretical advantages of SPECT imaging over planar imaging, including increased lesion contrast and the ability to define the size and number of defects more accurately. SPECT also improves sensitivity in the posterior myocardium. Thallium imaging should be viewed as complimentary to the ECG examination since the ECG measures different manifestations of myocardial ischemia. The two studies should not be compared, since thallium imaging is never done alone but in conjunction with the ECG. The gold standard for assessing sensitivity and specificity of exercise thallium scintigraphy has been the angiographic diagnosis of 50% narrowing of the diameter of a coronary artery. There may, however, be considerable disagreement as to interpretation of degree of narrowing, and the degree of stenosis may not correlate with the degree to which coronary blood flow reserve is impaired. When thallium perfusion defects occur in a setting of stenoses that are less than 50% but that are long or multiple, they may be assessed as false-positive, although flow reserve abnormalities may be present. In addition, flow reserve abnormalities may occur in patients with left ventricular hypertrophy or nonepicardial coronary artery disease such as that seen in diabetics. These abnormalities may be detected by thallium scintigraphy alone.

A number of factors affect the interpretation of the sensitivity and specificity of thallium scintigraphy in the diagnosis of coronary artery disease. The predictive accuracy of a test is dependent on the prevalence of the disease in the population that is tested. Thallium exercise testing is most helpful in patients who have an intermediate probability of coronary artery disease. Patients with a low probability of having coronary artery disease are not ideally suited to thallium scintigraphy. Also, in the scenario of high probability of coronary artery disease thallium scintigraphy should not be used solely for confirmation of disease. Some generalizations also apply to patients who have suffered myocardial infarctions. Submaximal stress testing before discharge is helpful in identifying survivors who remain at risk for future cardiac events. Thallium scintigraphy is also more helpful than exercise ECG in identifying patients with multivessel disease after infarction. Patients with prior infarctions who have been identified to be at high risk for future cardiac events need not necessarily have thallium scintigraphy for risk stratification. Posttherapy testing is sometimes helpful to determine whether therapy has depressed or masked ischemia. Occasionally, resting thallium imaging is done in patients with unstable coronary artery disease when redistribution is helpful to distinguish ischemic dysfunction from scar. Myocardial segments that show redistribution are thought to represent viable myocardium with a potential for revascularization.

Thallium scintigraphy should be particularly stressed for determination of prognosis. Findings that correlate with the risk of future cardiac events include the number and severity of reversible defects, defects in the left main coronary artery distribution, and abnormal lung uptake. Patients scheduled for vascular surgery who have no evidence of thallium redistribution on preoperative studies have a lower rate of perioperative cardiac events than patients who have redistribution. Patients with chest pain and no evidence of thallium redistribution have a cardiac event rate of approximately 1% per year. Several studies report cardiac event (infarction or death) rates of 1% or less following negative thallium scintigraphy studies. Dipyridamole thallium studies have also been useful for risk stratification after myocardial infarction. Abnormal scans with redistribution identify patients who are at significantly greater risk for future myocardial infarctions or sudden death. Overall, thallium scintigraphic studies have been demonstrated to have significant impact in studies where patient follow-up has been used as the gold standard for evaluation.

Brief mention should be made of the interpretive value of the worsening of thallium perfusion defects on delayed imaging or the visualization of defects only on rest images. This has been termed **reverse redistribution** and has no clear prognostic value (Fig. 2-10). The finding may be present in patients who have suffered a nontransmural infarction where there is a masking of the defect on stress imaging only. It has been theorized that peri-infarct hyperemia seen on stress images may account for this finding, but reverse redistribution may be present in patients with no evidence of coronary artery disease.

Some of the physical characteristics of thallium-201 make it a less than ideal radiopharmaceutical for cardiovascular imaging. The low-energy mercury x-rays result in significant attenuation and scatter, particularly in the obese patient. The 73-hour half-life of thallium-201 and distribution pattern within the body also results in less than ideal **dosimetry,** since the kidneys, gonads, and lens of the eye receive the highest dose. Administered doses are generally limited to 3 mCi, which results in a renal absorbed dose of 3.6 rad. Improved photon flux would result from use of a Tc-99m-labeled radiopharmaceutical, and this should at least theoretically improve the quality of SPECT images. Significant effort has therefore focused on development of three Tc-99m radiopharmaceuticals with significantly different physiologic properties. Tc-99m-sestamibi has become the preferred agent among the new isonitriles, and Tc-99m-teboroxime now represents the group of agents known as BATO compounds (boronic adducts of technetium oxime). Tc99m-tetrofosmin is a diphosphine cation that has been recently approved.

Tc-99m-sestamibi is a cation that diffuses into the

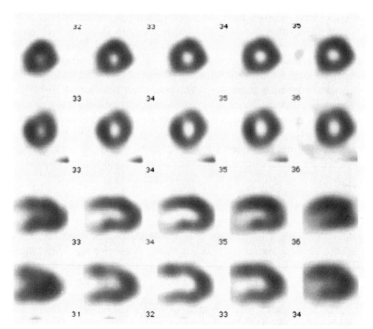

Figure 2-10. Reverse redistribution. Thallium-201 images in the short and sagittal axis following treadmill exercise (above) and following rest (below). Images following exercise are unremarkable but a defect appears in the anterior wall at rest. Reverse redistribution may be due to technical considerations and has no clear prognostic value.

myocardium relative to blood flow. Distribution underestimates blood flow at very high coronary flow rates. The major distinction between isonitriles such as sestamibi and the BATO compounds is that isonitriles have a much longer period of myocardial retention after injection. After injection of sestamibi, approximately 1 to 2% localizes within the myocardium. The myocardial half-life is approximately 6 hours after injection at rest. The biological half-life in the liver is approximately 30 minutes, and the major path for clearance of sestamibi is through the hepatobiliary system. Since the imaging time should be optimized for the relationship between myocardial and liver activity, images are generally obtained 1 hour after administration after the patient has consumed a glass of milk to facilitate emptying of the gall bladder (Fig. 2-11). A recent suggested improvement on this protocol is to image at 15 minutes after injection before hepatobiliary activity is a problem. Ingestion of milk is then not needed.

Because of the long myocardial retention time of sestamibi, a number of imaginative protocols have been developed to image patients on the same day. One popular protocol involves giving a smaller dose of sestamibi in the range of 8 to 10 mCi at rest followed by imaging 4 hours later at stress with a larger dose (20 to 30 mCi). Imaging is also delayed for 30 to 60 minutes follow-

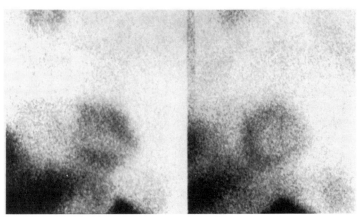

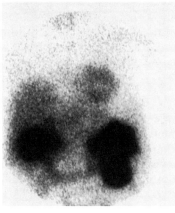

Figure 2-11. Infradiaphragmatic activity following Tc-99m-sestamibi injection. Anterior and LAO planar image and anterior body image following injection of 8 to 10 mCi of Tc-99m-sestamibi at rest. These early images were done intentionally to show the significant hepatic, biliary, and bowel excretion of sestamibi. Images should therefore be obtained 1 hour after administration of tracer and after the patient has consumed a glass of milk to facilitate emptying of the gall bladder. A good alternative is to image at 15 minutes before biliary activity is a problem.

ing injection. After injection approximately 33% of the administered sestamibi is cleared through the gastrointestinal tract and
27% is excreted in the urine.

The overall SPECT imaging protocol for sestamibi is similar
to that for thallium with use of a 180-degree rotation, typically
with 30 stops. The larger injected dose relative to thallium provides for more rapid acquisition of planar images prior to
SPECT acquisition. Another advantage of sestamibi is that
patients may be studied at significant intervals after injection. A
dose prepared for standby use can be given in the patient care
unit when symptoms arise. Imaging can be performed several
hours later. Since redistribution is minimal one injection will not
allow differentiation of viable from scarred myocardium.

Tc-99m-teboroxime belongs to the class of BATO agents.
Like thallium and sestamibi, teboroxime is rapidly cleared from
the blood following injection, with approximately 10% remaining within the blood at 10 minutes following injection. Also like
sestamibi, this agent is excreted predominantly through the
hepatobiliary system. The critical dose is to the proximal colon
and to a lesser extent gallbladder wall. After 24 hours urinary
excretion averages approximately 22%. Extremely rapid clearance from the myocardium distinguishes this neutral lipid-solu-
ble agent from sestamibi or thallium. After teboroxime peaks in
the myocardium at 3.5% of the injected dose, there is a rapid
biexponential clearance with half-life components of 6 minutes
and 13 hours. The overall biological half-life is in the 10- to 20-
minute range. This does not allow time for clearance of significant hepatic or gallbladder activity. Although planar images can
be obtained, special modifications must be made to allow
SPECT acquisition. The theoretical advantage of teboroxime is
that separate rest and stress examinations may be performed
within a period of less than 2 hours. At the present time use of
teboroxime is declining.

Tc-99m-tetrofosmin is the newest agent that is approved for
myocardial perfusion imaging. Like sestamibi, this agent shows
significant retention within the myocardium and no significant
redistribution. Recent studies have shown that myocardial
uptake is between 1 and 2% and that clearance from the blood
and liver is rapid. The highest dose is to the gallbladder wall.
Heating is not necessary for preparation. Good-quality SPECT
images can be obtained 15 minutes after injection. Early investi-

gations suggest sensitivity and specificity for coronary artery disease that is comparable to thallium imaging.

At the present time the only agent to show significant redistribution within the myocardium is thallium-201. The ultimate Tc-99m radiopharmaceutical will have physiologic properties similar to thallium with the benefit of increased photon flux. The technetium agents could theoretically improve imaging in patients where significant soft-tissue attenuation would be expected. Protocols for use of these agents are constantly being suggested and modified, and no ultimate protocol exists. Creative investigators are combining use of thallium-201 and Tc-99m-sestamibi or Tc99m-tetrofosmin in the same patient for a rest/stress evaluation at different photopeaks. Early interest in this **hybrid protocol** utilizing thallium-201 for rest imagimg and Tc-99m-sestamibi or tetrofosmin for exercise imaging focused on simultaneous acquisition of images at different photopeaks. It is now known that there is considerable scatter from Tc-99m into the thallium-201 window, which can degrade the contrast between normal and abnormal myocardium. Therefore a separate acquisition hybrid protocol has been developed to avoid the problem of cross talk between the different isotope windows. Three mCi of thallium-201 is injected at rest and SPECT imaging is begun 10 minutes after injection. Immediately after this acquisition the patient undergoes the exercise phase and receives 25 mCi of Tc-99m-sestamibi. SPECT imaging utilizing the Tc-99m window is then begun 15 minutes after injection. A 15% window centered on the 140keV Tc-99m photopeak reduces the effect of scatter. Since high-resolution collimators can be used for both the Tc-99m and thallium-201 acquisitions, there is an acceptable difference between image resolution of the rest and stress phases. This hybrid protocol is now finding more widespread application. A further modification of this hybrid protocol involves the injection of thallium-201 approximately 12 hours prior to rest imaging in order to further enhance the benefit of thallium redistribution.

Gated Blood Pool Imaging

The evaluation of left ventricular function and ejection fraction by first-pass and equilibrium technique has remained a mainstay of clinical nuclear medicine. **First-pass** evaluation of right or left ventricular ejection fraction is not as frequently obtained today as equilibrium gated blood pool imaging but is useful in selected circumstances. The premise is that ejection fraction can be adequately determined by the passage of a compact bolus through the right and then left sides of the heart. A compact injection of high specific activity can be obtained by placing an external jugular catheter, but this is rarely done. An antecubital vein can also be used in association with a blood pressure cuff. Use of pertechnetate is adequate unless multiple injections are planned. If multiple evaluations are needed, Tc-99m-DTPA is more useful, since it is rapidly cleared by the kidneys. Use of Tc-99m-sulfur colloid allows accumulation of activity within the liver and spleen, which may interfere with cardiac imaging. The use of Au-195m with its short half-life of 30.5 seconds has not been approved in the United States because of contamination by the parent nuclide. Once injection of pertechnetate has been made for first-pass evaluation, a single or multicrystal gamma camera can be employed to obtain images of several myocardial contractions. Specialized equipment that can handle count rates up to 500,000 per second was available in the 1970s and 1980s but is more difficult to obtain today. Single-crystal gamma cameras that show linear count rate responses up to 60,000 counts per second must therefore be utilized. This produces images that are of limited count density and limited spatial resolution. Ejection fraction calculation is also impeded by incomplete mixing of the injected bolus with the ventricular blood pool. The camera should be placed in the 30-degree right anterior oblique position to facilitate separation of the right ventricle from the right atrium. Typically, five or six beats of the right ventricle are incorporated for evaluation of ejection fraction. The subjective process of choosing the appropriate set of data from such a short sequence with limited count density has obscured the utility of this study. Therefore evaluation of ejection fraction and wall motion has generally given way to use of resting or exercise equilibrium gated blood pool imaging. However, the quantitation of left to right intracardiac shunts is still done with the first-pass technique.

Scintigraphic procedures can be helpful in the detection and quantitation of **left-to-right shunts** such as atrial and ventricular septal defects and patent ductus arteriosus. Normally, tracer passes through the right side of the heart, the lungs, and the left side of the heart, then there is a delay of 8 to 10 seconds before recirculation of tracer is again noted in the right side of the heart and pulmonary bed. An early recirculation of tracer can be detected by means of **Qp:Qs** (pulmonary flow:systemic flow) quantitation. If a region of interest is drawn over the peripheral portion of the lungs and images are framed at a rapid rate of 10 to 20 frames per second, a recirculation peak can be noted in the lung time–activity profile. A second region of interest is drawn over the superior vena cava to ensure that a compact bolus lasting less than 2 to 4 seconds is obtained. The lung region of interest is commonly drawn in the anterior projection over the right lung to avoid interference from cardiac blood pool activity. The time–activity curve of the lung region of interest is then best analyzed by the gamma variate function. Using this approach the initial pulmonary activity curve is fitted with a gamma variate function. The area under the recirculation peak is also fitted with a gamma variate function and the difference between the areas under the pulmonary and recirculation curves is proportional to the amount of shunted blood. The normal Qp:Qs ratio should be 1.0 and values above 1.2 should be considered abnormal. The most common cause of problems with the Qp:Qs technique is alteration of the time–activity curve by an inadequate bolus.

Another application of scintigraphic techniques is seen in patients with **right-to-left shunting.** Quantitation may be helpful for a number of clinical conditions, including Eisenmenger complex, severe pulmonary stenosis, tricuspid or pulmonary atresia, tetralogy of Fallot, transposition of the great vessels, and hepatogenic pulmonary angiodysplasia. A simple and reliable method involves intravenous injection Tc-99m-MAA particles. Either limited imaging of the thorax and head or total body quantitation of MAA distribution is useful. Since 90% of the MAA particles are between 10 and 90 μ, there should normally be limited visualization of the nonpulmonary capillary bed. When images of the head and thorax are obtained a general guideline is that activity in the head be limited to 2 to 3% of the thoracic activity (Fig. 2-12). Total body images give a more accurate representation of the absolute degree of shunting and can be useful in sequential follow-up when medical or surgical intervention has taken place.

Gated blood pool scanning is synonymous with multiple uptake gated acquisition (**MUGA**). There are several choices of

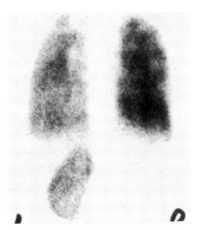

Figure 2-12. Right to left shunting. Posterior imaging of the thorax and upper abdomen following injection of Tc-99m-MAA intravenously reveals evidence of heterogeneous deposition of MAA within the lungs and right to left shunting to a solitary left kidney. Total body imaging could be used to quantitate the degree of shunting. Limited imaging of the thorax and abdomen or head and thorax can also be performed to estimate the degree of shunting.

radiopharmaceutical preparation. Tc-99m human serum albumin may be sufficient for a routine calculation of left ventricular ejection fraction prior to and after the onset of cardiotoxic chemotherapy. Although human serum albumin may be rapidly prepared for administration of multiple doses, there is a loss of image quality due to leakage of albumin to the extravascular space. Albumin is insufficient for use with gated acquisitions during exercise when target to background ratios become unacceptable. Images of better quality are achieved by one of three methods of labeling red blood cells (RBCs).

The **in vivo method** is the simplest way of labeling RBCs and produces labeling efficiencies in the 80 to 90% range. An unlabeled pyrophosphate kit is injected intravenously, supplying approximately 1 mg of stannous pyrophosphate as a reducing agent. After 20 minutes, 15 to 30 mCi of Tc-99m pertechnetate are injected intravenously. Pertechnetate diffuses into the RBCs, where reduction by stannous ion allows binding to the beta chain of hemoglobin. The pertechnetate that does not diffuse into the red cells binds nonspecifically to plasma proteins and diffuses into the extracellular fluid space, degrading overall image quality. A better method of labeling is the modified **in vivo method,** where the patient is again injected intravenously with a nonradioactive stannous pyrophosphate kit. After 20 minutes 2 to 10 mL of blood are withdrawn into a syringe and 15 to 30 minutes of pertechnetate is added. After 10 to 20 minutes the labeled blood sample is reinjected with a labeling efficiency of approximately 95%. The best method of labeling RBCs and a method that is recommended for exercise gated acquisitions and blood loss studies is the **in vitro method.** With this method labeling efficiencies are consistently greater than 95% . A small sample of 1 to 3 mL of whole blood are withdrawn into a vial containing stannous chloride and acid citrate dextrose as an anticoagulant. After approximately 5 minutes sodium hypochlorite is added to oxidize any stannous ion that remains extracellular. Fifteen to 30 mCi of pertechnetate are then added, allowing essentially only reduction of pertechnetate within the RBCs. Following an incubation period of 15 to 20 minutes the entire sample is injected intravenously. For all labeling methods there are some general considerations. Pertechnetate is known to label heparin, and therefore acid citrate dextrose (ACD) may be the preferable anticoagulant. As with other Tc-99m preparations, oxidation by exposure to room air should be avoided. Whenever possible stannous pyrophosphate should not be injected through an intravenous line. Other factors that interfere with RBC labeling include the recent administration of a variety of **antihypertensive agents,** presence of **digoxin,** and the presence of **sickle cell hemoglobin** or **RBC antibodies.**

Image acquisition is performed using R wave triggering and division of the R-R interval into 16 to 32 frames. Repeat acquisition of the R-R interval continues until approximately 150,000 to 500,000 counts are achieved per frame. The most common method is frame mode acquisition using a 20% window for R-R interval length. If an aberrant interval is detected, the following one or two intervals can be rejected. This would eliminate some aberrant beats in patients with bigeminy or trigeminy. An alternate method for rejecting aberrant beats involves on-the-fly analysis by interim storage of R-R intervals within a buffer. In patients where ectopic beats represents up to 20 or 30% of all collected data, list mode acquisition becomes the most rigorous method. All data are stored and written to a disk file. Beat length windowing is not attempted. Instead a histogram is created for R-R intervals of various durations. The R-R intervals with greatest frequency can then be selected to produce the gated image. List mode acquisition is generally reserved for patients with relatively severe dysrhythmias. All conditions associated with R-R interval variability or with altered P, R, or T wave amplitude will degrade image acquisition. No technique entirely eliminates the influence of an abnormal cardiac contraction on subsequent contractions.

Image acquisition of the gated study is performed with either a standard- or large-field-of-view gamma camera. A zoom factor of 1.5 may be necessary with a larger-field-of-view camera. An all-purpose or high-resolution low-energy collimator is sufficient at rest, whereas a high-sensitivity collimator will provide more counts during exercise. One factor that has a significant influence is the positioning of the gamma camera relative to the patient. Optimal angulation can be achieved when there is good separation of the right and left ventricular blood pools. Slight caudal angulation can be useful to separate left ventricular and left atrial blood pool activity. The anterior and left lateral views are generally obtained after the LAO 45 degree view. SPECT acquisition of gated blood pool studies is possible for infrequent applications. Reconstruction provides images that are oriented in the short axis and sagittal long axis. Slant-hole collimators have been developed to provide a better separation of the ventricular and atrial blood pools.

Reconstruction of the gated blood pool study includes temporal and spatial smoothing of data. The background region of interest should be carefully checked by the technologist since it can drastically affect the calculation of **ejection fraction.** The formula for calculation of LVEF is the background-corrected stroke volume divided by the background-corrected endiastolic counts. A high background will falsely increase the ejection fraction and is a common cause of errors. Care should be taken that the blood pool of the atrium, ventricle, aorta or spleen are not included in the background region of interest. A normal LVEF is 50 to 65% and a normal RVEF is 45 to 60%.

A number of algorithms have been applied to calculate the boundaries of the endiastolic and endsystolic blood pools. These include use of the first and second derivatives of the count rate profiles. Any automated or semiautomated technique should always be checked by visual examination of the study. The error for calculation of the left ventricular ejection fraction is in the one- to two-point range for near normal levels but may increase to five points or greater for very low ejection fractions. Errors of right ventricular ejection fraction are significantly greater because of limited separation of the right ventricular and right atrial blood pools. A complete visual assessment for wall motion includes examination of the anterior, LAO, and left lateral acquisitions. Significant inward motion of the inferoapical and lateral walls should be seen on the LAO 45-degree projection. There is a lesser contribution from the septum. The anterior wall and apex are better seen in the anterior view. Examination of the inferior wall is optimized in the left lateral projection. The greater volume of the right ventricle relative to the left ventricle should be apparent.

The terms *hypokinetic* (decreased), *akinetic* (absent), *tardikinetic* (delayed), and *dyskinetic* are appropriate (Fig. 2-13). Dyskinesia of the septum is usually referred to as paradoxical septal motion. Sensitivity for detection of focal dyskinetic zones is reasonable, but specific interpretation of the presence of an aneurysm or pseudoaneurysm is limited. Photon-deficient impressions from the papillary muscles can occasionally be seen in the left ventricular blood pool. A pericardial effusion or significant thickening of the myocardium can often be detected. Implantable cardiac defibrillator patches or other hardware can occasionally alter the appearance of the left ventricular blood pool. A common occurrence on cine loop examination is the presence of count dropoff at the end of the averaged R-R interval. This may be present with increased R-R variability, and can cause significant count loss during display. Deletion of the final frames in the cine display is often an option with viewing software and can be helpful.

A number of quantitative computer methods can also occasionally be helpful. When the end-systolic image is subtracted from the end-diastolic image, a stroke volume image is obtained. If the diastolic image is subtracted from the systolic image, an inverse stroke volume image or paradox image can be obtained and can identify dyskinetic segments. Most helpful is the use of **Fourier transformation** to show **phase analysis.** Individual pixels or small groups of pixels in the ventricles should rise and fall in phase with each other. The atria should be 180 degrees out of phase with the ventricles. Phase analysis can help in detection of the atrioventricular boundaries. Abnormal phase analysis would be expected at sites of premature activation in Wolff-Parkinson-White syndrome. Left bundle branch block would result in delayed phase of the left ventricle. Any dyskinetic or tardikinetic myocardial segment will appear to be out of phase with the left

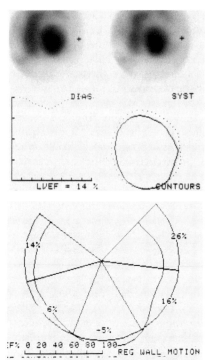

Figure 2-13. Gated blood pool study. End-diastolic and end-systolic images from a gated radionuclide ventriculogram reveal a dilated left ventricle, a markedly decreased ejection fraction, diffuse hypokinesis, and slight apical dyskinesis by regional wall motion analysis.

of the ventricle and will be assigned a shade of gray or color that is different from the remainder of the left ventricular blood pool. Proper examination of a gated blood pool includes examination of the phase analysis on the hard copy followed by visual review of the cine display.

There are a number of applications of resting gated blood pool imaging. A frequent application in today's clinical practice is seen in patients who are receiving **doxorubicin (Adriamycin).** The effects of doxorubicin toxicity may appear when a cumulative dose of 350 mg/m^2 has been administered. Up to one-third of patients may develop cardiotoxicity at doses greater than 550 mg/m^2. A gated blood pool study is often performed prior to chemotherapy or when the cumulative dose approaches 300 mg/m^2. Moderate cardiotoxicity is defined as a drop in the left ventricular ejection fraction of greater than 15 points or an absolute left ventricular ejection fraction of less than 45%. At this point doxorubicin administration may be discontinued and the patient may be studied at a later date. In selected cases an exercise gated blood pool examination may be performed to assess left ventricular reserve in patients who have had a drop in ejection fraction. If left ventricular reserve is adequate, doxorubicin therapy may occasionally be continued.

Resting gated blood pool studies are occasionally performed in patients with recent myocardial infarctions (Fig. 2-14). The prognosis of the patient is linked to the degree of functional impairment of the left ventricle, and prognosis is worse when serial ejection fraction studies show declining function. Exercise gated blood pool studies may occasionally be useful for evaluating patients with coronary artery disease. An abnormal exercise study would be one in which ejection fraction units do not rise by at least five points (Fig. 2-15). A fall in ejection fraction would be a more specific indicator, but absence of an increase of ejection fraction during exercise also provides evidence of coronary artery disease. The overall sensitivity of exercise gated blood pool studies for coronary artery disease is approximately 85%. Because noncoronary heart disease may also manifest as a drop in ejection fraction during exercise, the specificity of the study is limited. A significant number of older or female patients may normally show no increase in left ventricular ejection fraction during exercise. In these individuals increases in end-diastolic volumes may contribute more significantly to cardiac output than increases in ejection fraction.

Valvular heart disease is another indication for gated blood pool imaging. The stroke volume ratio of the ventricles should be 1.0, but left ventricular stroke volume may rise with aortic or mitral regurgitation. Left ventricular to right ventricular stroke volume ratios should rise with greater degrees of aortic or mitral regurgitation. A decrease in left ventricular end-diastolic volume during exercise indicates functional abnormality of the left ventricle in a patient with valvular heart disease.

Evaluation of patients with hypertrophic cardiomyopathies is typically done with echocardiography. Diastolic filling would be expected to be abnormal in this population, and ejection fractions can be elevated because of the small left ventricular chamber size. In patients with congestive cardiomyopathies the left ventricle is typically dilated and diffusely dysfunctional with hypokinesis, tardikinesis or dyskinesis of multiple myocardial

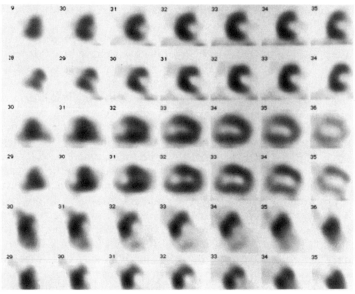

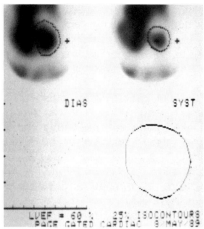

Figure 2-14. Lateral wall infarct. Dipyridamole SPECT with thallium-201 imaging in three orientations with stress images above and rest images below. After reinjection with thallium-201 there is a persistent lateral photopenic defect compatible with a myocardial infarct. Gated blood pool study reveals a normal left ventricular ejection fraction of 60% with lateral wall akinesis.

segments. The phase analysis image is often diffusely abnormal. With coronary artery disease a specific coronary artery distribution may be impaired. Drug therapy can be monitored by changes in ejection fraction and wall motion. Patients awaiting heart transplantation are typically assessed with resting gated

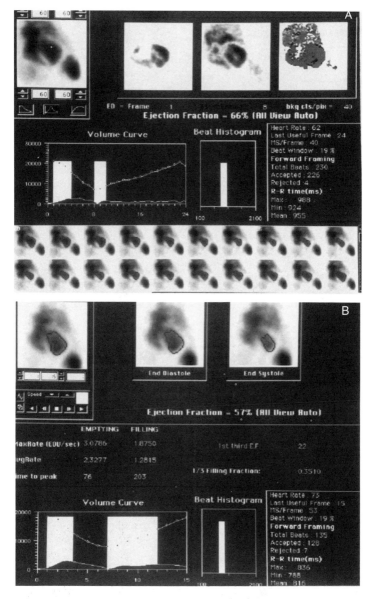

Figure 2-15. *continued*

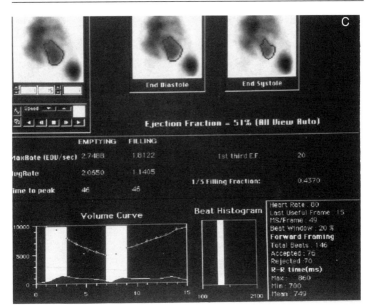

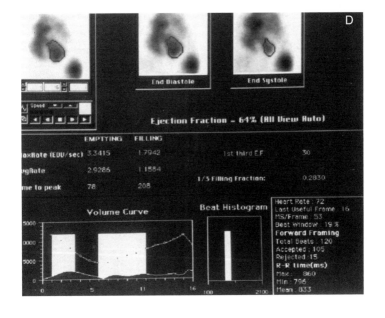

Figure 2-15. *(pages 37 and 38)* Exercise gated blood pool study. This patient, who had a history of aortic valvular insufficiency, was studied at rest, during treadmill exercise stages 1 and 2, and immediately after exercise. Note the moderate left ventricular dilation. The study also revealed an abnormal fall in ejection fraction from 66 to 57%, and further to 51% during exercise stage 2. The patient showed recovery to a left ventricular ejection fraction of 64% during the postexercise phase. The exercise stages were performed at 3-minute intervals, and 2 minutes of each interval were used for image acquisition. Note the abnormal drop in end-diastolic counts during exercise.

blood pool imaging in the preoperative period. Another application of resting blood pool imaging is in patients with pulmonary disease. Abnormal right ventricular dilation and abnormal wall motion may be seen in patients with long-standing pulmonary hypertension. Estimates of right ventricular ejection fraction are limited by the overlap of the right atrial and right ventricular blood pools. Errors are seen when the right atrial end-diastolic volume overlaps the right ventricular end-systolic volume, leading to underestimation of right ventricular ejection fraction.

Infarct Imaging

Infarct avid imaging is a procedure that is not commonly performed in today's clinical practice. In selected circumstances when history, CK-MB fractions, or the ECG are not specific, imaging with **Tc-99m-pyrophosphate** can be useful. The diagnosis of myocardial infarction may be uncertain in these patients because of the timing after suspected infarction or because of the patient's postoperative state. Although uptake of pyrophosphate may be seen as early as 4 hours after coronary artery occlusion, the highest sensitivity for myocardial infarction is obtained between 48 and 72 hours after the suspected myocardial event (Fig. 2-16). Sensitivity for a non-transmural infarction is approximately 80%, and the detection rate for transmural infarction is higher. SPECT is occasionally useful to localize and size the area of infarction. After direct intravenous injection of 20 mCi of Tc-99m-pyrophosphate, images of at least 400,000 counts are typically obtained in the anterior, 30 degrees LAO, 60 degrees LAO, and left lateral projections (Fig. 2-17). Imaging is usually obtained at 3 to 4 hours following injection. Uptake of pyrophosphate is graded on a scale of 0 to 4+, where 2+ would indicate definite myocardial accumulation at an intensity slightly less than bone, and 4+ would indicate intense uptake greater than bone. Studies are judged to be positive when intensity is at least 2+. The great majority of infarctions involve the anterior wall or septum. Inferior or posterior septal activity is less commonly seen. The right ventricle may occasionally be involved when the left ventricular inferior wall is positive. An ominous finding is the doughnut type of accumulation pattern with a central area of absent perfusion. The mechanism of uptake is thought to be pyrophosphate binding to calcium phosphate in either the amorphous or hydroxyapatite forms. Calcium influx is seen when there has been significant myocardial damage, and pyrophosphate accumulation may therefore be seen following cardioversion or major surgery or trauma. Diffuse right and left ventricular uptake is seen in patients with cardiac amyloidosis (Fig. 2-18).

In-111-labeled antimyosin Fab fragments have been injected to localize and quantitate areas of necrotic myocardium. Sensitivity is highest at approximately 24 to 48 hours following infarction. Uptake is due to disruption of the myocardial cell membrane with exposure of myosin to the radiopharmaceutical. In-111-antimyosin has also been advocated for evaluation of heart trans-

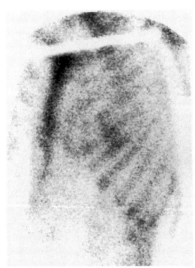

Figure 2-16. Infarct imaging. Abnormal left ventricular uptake of Tc-99-m-pyrophosphate is seen 48 hours after a suspected septal infarction. The intensity of pyrophosphate accumulation on this LAO view is slightly greater than that of the ribs and less than that of the sternum. Uptake would thus be approximately 3+ on a scale of 0 to 4+. Images are usually obtained 3 to 4 hours after PYP injection.

Figure 2-17. Lateral wall myocardial infarction. Intense pyrophosphate accumulation is seen in the anterior, 30 degrees LAO, 60 degrees LAO, and left lateral projections. Multiple views obtained with 400,000 or 500,000 counts each are useful for infarct localization.

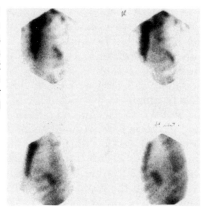

plant recipients during acute rejection episodes. These applications of antimyosin imaging have not found widespread acceptance.

Positron Emission Tomography

Positron emission tomography (PET) may be the most promising tool for evaluation of myocardial perfusion and metabolism, but is at present limited by cost and lack of availability. **Rubidium-82** is a perfusion tracer that is available from a strontium-82 generator. Its short half-life of 76 seconds allows serial blood flow mea-

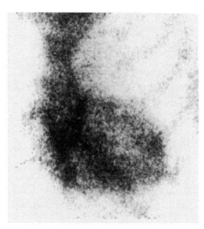

Figure 2-18. Cardiac amyloidosis. Diffuse intense biventricular myocardial uptake may be seen with cardiac amyloidosis. Some other uncommon causes of diffuse activity include pericarditis or myocarditis, cardiotoxicity secondary to radiation or Adriamycin, or trauma following cardioversion.

surements. Other PET radiopharmaceuticals are cyclotron produced and have a short half-life mandating that a cyclotron facility be available for most types of examinations. **Oxygen-15** is used as a perfusion tracer in the form of oxygen-15 water, has a half-life of 2 minutes, and shows rapid equalization with surrounding soft tissues. **Nitrogen-13** is used in the form of nitrogen-13 ammonia, has a half-life of 10 minutes, and shows good myocardial-to-background ratios based on myocardial extraction and retention in the form of glutamine. **Fluorine-18** is used as fluorine-18-FDG (fludeoxyglucose), has a half-life of 110 minutes, and reflects the shift from long-chain fatty acids to glucose as a myocardial substrate during ischemia. Patients may be studied with PET in the resting state following dipyridamole or adenosine infusion. Sites of decreased blood flow in conjunction with decreased uptake of fluorine-18-FDG suggest the presence of scar. Sites of decreased perfusion in conjunction with uptake of fluorine-18-FDG suggest the presence of viable myocardium and a potential for revascularization (Fig. 2-19). The overall sensitivity and specificity of PET for diagnosis of coronary artery disease is greater than 90%. There is some benefit of PET imaging over thallium SPECT imaging for detection of coronary artery disease, but the benefit is minimized when thallium reinjection protocols are used. PET imaging retains an advantage in differentiation viable from scarred myocardium. Only rarely do cardiac segments that show no FDG accumulation demonstrate functional improvement following revascularization. The image quality of PET studies is high because of the general lack of soft-tissue attenuation artifacts.

Lymphoscintigraphy

Lymphoscintigraphy is a safe and easy procedure that allows differentiation of causes of **lymphedema** and also maps lymphatic drainage patterns of **melanoma** and other tumors. Early studies used gold colloids that produced unacceptable radiation doses to the injection sites. Since the 1970s various materials have been labeled with Tc-99m. Recently, Tc-99m **antimony trisulfide colloid** was the preferred material, with a particle size of 30 to 120A. This product is presently not available. The two best choices for radiopharmaceutical currently are human serum albumin and sulfur colloid. **Human serum albumin** is adequate

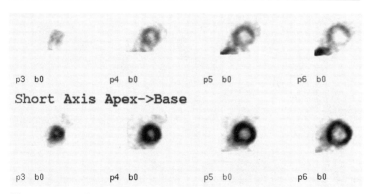

p3 b0   p4 b0   p5 b0   p6 b0

Short Axis Apex->Base

p3 b0   p4 b0   p5 b0   p6 b0

Figure 2-19. Positron emission tomography. This is a combined study using N-13 ammonia for assessment of perfusion (top) and F-18 fludeoxyglucose for assessment of myocardial glucose uptake. Although there is abnormally decreased inferoapical perfusion, evidence of glucose uptake can be seen. This suggests the potential for revascularization in this patient. (Courtesy of Donald S. Schauwecker, M.D., Ph.D., Indiana University Medical Center, Indianapolis, Indiana.)

for both lymphedema evaluation and tumor drainage studies. The only disadvantage is that albumin is not retained in significant amounts within the lymph nodes. Albumin is therefore most useful for study of lymphedema. **Sulfur colloid** can be used, because it has a particle size in the range of 0.1 to 1.0 µm (85%), with a mean size of approximately 0.3 µm. Sulfur colloid is well suited to tumor drainage studies and can be optimized with filtration through a 0.1- or 0.2- µm filter. Sulfur microcolloid with a particle size of less than .05 µm can also be used. For evaluation of lymphedema, 1 to 3 mCi of Tc-99m human serum albumin in 0.1 to 0.2 mL are injected into each of four web sites in the hands or feet. Injection should be into the dermal or subdermal interstitium using a 23- or 25-gauge needle. The patient can be studies every 30 minutes up to approximately 4 to 6 hours. Collateral patterns of drainage such as the dermal backflow pattern suggest occluded or nonexistent deep lymphatic channels. Occasionally, a level of obstruction can be determined by the pattern of collateral drainage (Figs. 2-20 and 2-21).

The most frequent application of lymphoscintigraphy to oncology is determination of lymphatic drainage patterns of melanoma.

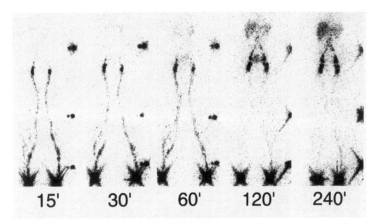

Figure 2-20. Normal lymphoscintigraphy study of the lower extremities. There is prompt and symmetric visualization of deep lymphatic channels in both lower extremities. A small amount of collateral flow is seen below the knee on the right, but the primary deep lymphatic channel is evident throughout.

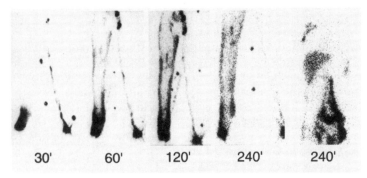

Figure 2-21. Congenital lymphedema of right lower extremity. A stocking-like pattern of dermal collateral flow is seen on the right side with absence of a deep lymphatic channel and nonvisualization of the right-sided inguinal nodes. Lymphatic flow on the left is normal. Anterior abdominal view is seen at 240 minutes.

Circumferential injections of filtered sulfur colloid are used to detect either a sentinel node or a group of nodes at risk for metastatic involvement. Although this study is occasionally useful for detection of sentinel nodes for breast cancer, internal mammary nodes are now infrequently evaluated by lymphoscintigraphy.

Suggested Reading

Beller GA: Myocardial perfusion imaging with Thallium-201. *J Nucl Med* 1994; 35:674-680.

Berman DS, Mosen SK, VanTrain KF, Germano G, Maddahi J, Friedman JD: Myocardial perfusion imaging with Tc99m-sestamibi: comparative analysis of available imaging protocols. *J Nucl Med* 1994; 35:681-688.

Bonow RO, Dilsizian V: Thallium-201 for assessment of myocardial viability. *Semin Nucl Med* 1991; 21:230-241.

Botvinick EH, Dae MW: Dipyridamole perfusion scintigraphy. *Semin Nucl Med* 1991; 21:242-265.

Brown KA. The role of stress redistribution thallium-201 myocardial perfusion imaging in evaluating coronary artery disease and perioperative risk. *J Nucl Med* 1994; 35:703-706.

Clements IP, Gibbons RJ, Mankin HT, Zinmeister AR, Brown ML: Guidelines for the interpretation of the exercise radionuclide ventriculogram for diagnosing coronary artery disease. *Am J Cardiol* 1987; 60:1265-1268.

Croll MN, Brady LW, Dadparar S: Implications of lymphoscintigraphy in oncologic practice. *Semin Nucl Med* 1983; 13:4.

DePuey EG: How to detect and avoid myocardial perfusion artifacts. *J Nucl Med* 1994; 35:699-702.

DePuey EG, Garcia EV: Optimal specificity of thallium-201 SPECT through recognition of imaging artifacts. *J Nucl Med* 1989;30:441.

Freeman LM, Blaufox MD, ed: Cardiovascular nuclear medicine. *Semin Nucl Med* 1991; 21.

Hurwitz RA, Treves ST: Nuclear cardiology. In: Adams FH, Emmanovilides GC., eds. *Moss' Heart Disease in Infants, Children and Adolescents*, 3rd ed. Baltimore: Williams and Wilkins, 1983; 101-107.

Iskandrian AS: Adenosine myocardial perfusion imaging. *J Nucl Med* 1994; 35:734-736.

Johnson LL: Myocardial perfusion imaging with technetium-99m teboroxime. *J Nucl Med* 1994; 35:689-692.

Leppo JA: Dipyridamole myocardial perfusion imaging. *J Nucl Med* 1994; 35:730-733.

Leppo JA: DePuey EG, Johnson LJ. A review of cardiac imaging with sestamibi and teboroxime. *J Nucl Med* 1991; 32:2012-2022.

Maddahi J, Schelbert H, Bronken R, DiCarli M: Role of thallium-201 and PET imaging in evaluation of myocardial viability and management of patients with coronary artery disease and left ventricular dysfunction. *J Nucl Med* 1994; 35:707-715.

Port SC: The role of radionuclide ventriculography in the assessment of prognosis in patients with CAD. *J Nucl Med* 1994; 35:721-725.

Rijke AM, Croft BY, Johnson RA, de Jongste AB, Camps JAJ: Lymphoscintigraphy and lyphedema of the lower extremities. *J Nucl Med* 1990; 31:990-998.

Ritchie JL, et al: Antracycline cardiotoxicity: clinical and pathologic outcomes assessed by radionuclide ejection fraction. Cancer 1980; 46:1109-1116.

Rocco TP, Dilsizian V, Fishman AJ, Strauss HW: Evaluation of ventricular function in patients with coronary artery disease. *J Nucl Med* 1989; 30:1149-1165.

Schwaiger M: Myocardial perfusion imaging with PET. *J Nucl Med* 1994; 35:693-698.

Schwaiger M, Hutchins GD: Evaluation of coronary artery disease with positron emission tomography. *Semin Nucl Med* 1992; 21:210.

Strauss HW, Boucher CA: Myocardial perfusion studies: lessons from a decade of clinical use. *Radiology* 1986; 160:577-584.

Verani MS: Dobutamine myocardial perfusion imaging. *J Nucl Med* 1994; 35:737-739.

Verani MS: Exercise and pharmacologic stress testing for prognosis of acute myocardial infarction. *J Nucl Med* 1994; 35:716-720.

Wackers FJTh. Exercise myocardial perfusion imaging. J. Nucl. Med. 35:726-729, 1994.

Witte CL, Witte MH: Discoders of lymph flow. *Acad Radiol 1995;* 2:234-334.

Chapter 3

Endocrine

Thyroid Diagnosis

Radiopharmaceuticals And Instrumentation

The radiotracers that are usually used to image the thyroid are I-131, I-123, and Tc-99m pertechnetate. Iodine is trapped by the thyroid and organified, and pertechnetate is trapped but not organified. Iodine may be preferable because it is more physiologic than pertechnetate and because it has higher iodine target-to-background ratios, but both I-131 and I-123 have significant disadvantages. I-131 is relatively inexpensive, but its 8-day half-life and beta radiation result in a high patient radiation dose. Furthermore, the predominant photon energy is 364 keV, higher than optimum for the gamma camera. I-123 has nearly ideal half-life and photon energy (13 hours and 159 keV), but it is expensive. Pertechnetate is very inexpensive, and imaging with this agent can be performed 20 to 40 minutes after injection, compared with several hours for iodine. However, because pertechnetate is not organified, images do not reflect the thryoid's ability to organify.

Images of optimum spatial resolution are obtained when the gamma camera is used with a pin-hole collimator, although high-quality images can be obtained with parallel-hole or converging collimators. Imaging can detect nonpalpable lesions that are somewhat less than 1 cm in diameter. Radioactive markers can be used in the image as landmarks for localization of palpable lesions.

Several exogenous materials can interfere with thyroid imaging. Iodine, either dietary or in radiographic contrast media, can significantly decrease uptake. Imaging should be delayed until 1 to 3 weeks after intravenous contrast administration. Antithyroid drugs such as propylthiouracil should be discontinued 1 week before imaging. Therapeutic T3 and T4 should be discontinued 2 weeks and 4 to 6 weeks, respectively, before imaging.

Tl-201 has been used for thyroid imaging in the setting of known or suspected thyroid cancer. Thallium accumulates not only in vascular lesions such as cancers, but also in benign vascular lesions such as some adenomas and thyroiditis. The sensitivity of thallium in cancer detection is high, but its specificity is low. The specificity can be improved through the use of delayed imaging, because thallium is retained longer in malignant than in benign lesions. Tl-201 may be useful in following patients with known differentiated thyroid carcinoma. This tracer has the advantage that thyroid hormone replacement need not be withdrawn from patients undergoing scintigraphy, and sensitivity is at least as high as for I-131 scintigraphy. Thallium-201 is significantly less sensitive than I-131 in the detection of normal residual thyroid tissue in patients who have undergone thyroidectomy.

Diffuse Disease

In the **multinodular thyroid** gland, focal regions of colloid cystic change, hyperplasia, and fibrosis are interspersed with normal thyroid tissue. If the gland becomes enlarged, the term multinodular goiter is appropriate. Scintigraphy shows multiple cold regions sometimes corresponding to palpable nodules interspersed with areas of normal to increased uptake (Fig. 3–1). This tissue showing increased uptake is autonomous;, that is, it has high uptake and produces increased T3 and T 4 even when thyroid-stimulating hormone (TSH) levels are low. This excessive T3 and T4 production by the autonomous tissue may result in clinical hyperthyroidism. The incidence of carcinoma in patients with multiple cold nodules in multinodular thyroid is about 1 to 6%, compared with 10 to 15% in patients with a solitary cold nodule in an otherwise normal thyroid gland. Ultrasound may be useful in establishing the diagnosis of multinodular thyroid when the nodules are too small to be detected by scintigraphy.

In **Graves' disease** (diffuse toxic goiter) an abnormal circulating autoantibody known as thyroid-stimulating antibody causes the thyroid to produce excessive amounts of T3 and T4. The etiology of the autoantibody formation is unknown, but infectious agents, mental stress, and genetic factors have been implicated.

Figure 3–1. Multinodular goiter (I-123) (anterior). The gland is enlarged and distorted by multiple nodules that have both decreased and increased uptake.

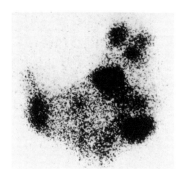

Scintigraphy with Tc-99m-pertechnetate or I-123 shows diffusely increased intensity relative to background in a gland that is anatomically normal except for enlargement (Fig. 3–2). A pyramidal lobe may be seen more frequently than in the normal thyroid. The percentage uptake of I-123 or I-131 is greater than 30% at 24 hours. The uptake is measured by comparing the count rate from the iodine dose in a neck phantom with the decay-corrected count rate of the patient's neck at 24 hours. Uptake is usually determined also at 4 hours, as a few patients with Graves's disease and other forms of hyperthyroidism show abnormal uptake at 4 hours but normal or decreased uptake at 24 hours.

Diffuse thyroiditis can be subacute or chronic. In **subacute thyroiditis** (de Quervain's disease) the relatively sudden onset of neck pain is followed by clinical hyperthyroidism. The incidence

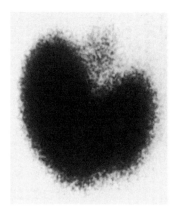

Figure 3–2. Graves' disease (T_cO_4) (anterior). The gland is enlarged and shows increased uptake relative to surrounding tissues. The pyramidal lobe is more prominent than usual.

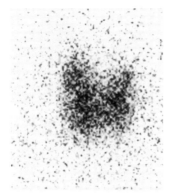

Figure 3–3. Subacute thyroiditis (I-123) (anterior). The gland appears anatomically normal but has decreased uptake (2% at 24 hours).

in women is five times that in men. This disease is probably caused by a virus that damages the thyroid tissue, resulting in discharge of thyroid hormones into the bloodstream and hyperthyroidism. The combination of damaged thyroid tissue and low TSH caused by the increased circulating thyroid hormone levels leads to decreased iodine uptake by the gland (Fig. 3–3). The process is usually diffuse and may be focal. In the ensuing weeks, the gland heals and the situation gradually returns to normal, sometimes with a period of hypothyroidism before healing is complete.

Chronic (Hashimoto's) thyroiditis is an autoimmune disease characterized by chronic inflammation, goiter with fine nodularity, and a long time course frequently leading to hypothyroidism. Almost all patients have circulating antithyroglobulin or antimicrosomal antibodies. These antibodies are also frequently detected in patients with Grave's disease. Women are affected four times more frequently than men. Variable timing of (1) release of T3 and T4 into the bloodstream because of tissue damage, (2) decreased thyroid function resulting from tissue damage, and (3) variable TSH levels reflecting changes causes unpredictable findings of clinical thyroid function and iodine uptake. Iodine scintigraphy may show increased or decreased uptake and variable degrees of nodularity and inhomogeneity.

Iodine-induced thyrotoxicosis (Jod–Basedow disease) is hyperthyroidism caused by high dietary iodine in susceptible patients. Imaging typically shows decreased uptake and nodularity.

Exogenous thyroid hormone, often taken factitiously in an

attempt to lose weight, is a cause of clinical hyperthyroidism. Because TSH levels are depressed by the excess circulating T3 and T4, imaging shows decreased uptake.

Focal Process

Solitary thyroid nodules discovered on scintigraphy are characterized as functioning or nonfunctioning. Functioning tissue can concentrate enough iodine tracer that this uptake can be detected on scintigraphy and can represent normal thyroid tissue, adenoma (Fig. 3–4), focal hyperplasia, or, very rarely, differentiated thyroid carcinoma. Functioning tissue can be further classified as autonomous or not autonomous. Autonomous tissue produces thyroid hormones independent of blood TSH levels. A nodule without detectable uptake of radioiodine may be a cyst, adenoma, abscess, or carcinoma (Fig. 3–5). Approximately 10 to 15% of cold nodules are carcinomas. An occasional nodule will show disparity between pertechnetate and iodine imaging. Because a rare cancer will be hot on pertechnetate imaging but cold on iodine imaging, some authorities have recommended that all hot nodules found with pertechnetate imaging should be reimaged with iodine to determine if they are cold in iodine images.

Of the benign solitary nodules, simple cysts may be differentiated from solid lesions effectively with ultrasound. Adenomas, which are usually nonfunctioning, are the commonest cause of cold nodules. Thyroid abscesses are associated with impressive clinical findings that make this diagnosis easy to differentiate from other cold nodules.

Of the 10 to 15% of cold nodules that are malignant (Table 3–1), about 80% are **differentiated thyroid cancer.** This classification includes papillary and follicular histologies. Both types tend to be indolent, and the papillary carcinomas are somewhat more benign than follicular. Many of these tumors contain histologic evidence of both architectures. A very rare differentiated thyroid cancer will produce enough thyroid hormone to cause hyperthyroidism, but the vast majority of these tumors produce very little thyroid hormone and take up little iodine tracer. **Anaplastic carcinoma** sometimes develops from differentiated carcinoma. This tumor grows rapidly and has a poor prognosis. **Medullary carcinoma** is intermediate in its behavior between differentiated and anaplastic tumors.

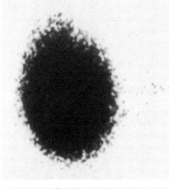

Figure 3–4. Autonomous nodule (T_cO_4) (anterior). This adenoma made the patient hyperthyroid. The resulting low TSH level has greatly reduced the uptake of the normal thyroid tissue.

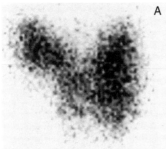

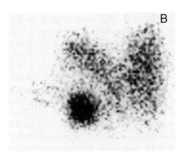

Figure 3–5. Cold nodule (I-123), without **(A)** and with **(B)** marker at the nodule (anterior). This was a differentiated carcinoma.

Thyroid cancer is associated with a history of therapeutic levels of radiation to the head and neck. Of patients with prior neck irradiation, 20 to 27% have thyroid nodules, not always solitary, and about one-third of patients with nodular thyroids and previous radiation have thyroid cancer.

Thyroid imaging is useful in the localization of **aberrant thyroid tissue** (Fig. 3–6). Aberrant thyroid tissue is sometimes not as tracer-avid or as productive of T3 and T4 as normally located tissue. Furthermore, iodine isotopes are concentrated in aberrant tissue more reliably than is pertechnetate. Anterior mediastinal goiter accounts for about 10% of mediastinal masses and can often be distinguished from other masses with iodine imaging. A rare cause of hyperthyroidism is struma ovarii, which is characterized by autonomous functioning thyroid tissue in an ovarian teratoma.

Table 3–1. Thyroid Cancers

Histology	Incidence(%)	Behavior	I-131 Uptake
Differentiated			
Papillary	62	Relatively benign	+*
Follicular	18	Less benign	+
Medullary	6	Intermediate	−
Anaplastic	14	Very malignant	−

*I-131 uptake in papillary carcinomas may depend on the presence of coexisting regions of follicular histology. The uptake is observed only when TSH levels are high.

I-131 Therapy

The beta radiation of I-131 causes a relatively high radiation dose to the thyroid gland in patients receiving this isotope. This radiation dose makes I-131 ideal for treating hyperthyroidism caused by Graves' disease or toxic nodular goiter. In these conditions, much of the radiation the patient receives is concentrated in the thyroid gland. The beta particles travel very short distances (several millimeters) in tissue, so structures near the thyroid are not affected significantly by the radiation. A treated toxic nodule, for example, is likely to respond to I-131, and surrounding normal thyroid tissue and the parathyroids are unlikely to be damaged.

Several formulas exist that yield the appropriate dose of therapeutic I-131 to be given to patients with Graves' disease. The

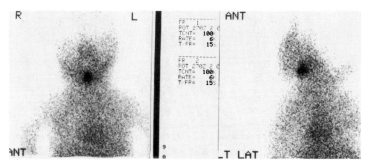

Figure 3–6. Lingual thyroid (I-123) (anterior, left, and left lateral, right). The only detectable thyroid tissue in this 16-month-old hypothyroid girl is at the base of the tongue.

desired administered dose can be calculated from thyroid gland weight, percent uptake at 24 hours, thyroidal turnover rate, and serum level of protein-bound I-131. Most formulas, however, yield the desired administered dose from gland weight, percent uptake at 24 hours, and desired radiation level. Any formula is inexact to some extent. Higher doses result in more cures but higher frequencies of eventual hypothyroidism. A useful simple formula is:

$D = (W/U) \times 10$, where D = dose of I-131 in millicuries, W = weight of the thyroid in grams, and U = percent 24 hour uptake.

In a patient with an average response to thyroid radiation, this formula yields a dose that is near the middle of the acceptable range. Half of the dose given by this formula would be near the lower end of the acceptable range and would result in fewer cures but in fewer eventual cases of hypothyroidism.

Following administration of I-131 for Graves' disease, euthyroidism is achieved gradually over a period of weeks to months. In the ensuing years, a significant fraction of treated patients will become hypothyroid. This phenomenon results from both the natural history of Graves' disease and the radiation-induced damage to the thyroid gland. Roughly one-third to one-half of the treated population eventually become hypothyroid.

The treatment of the autonomous functioning nodule requires a radiation dose that is several times higher than that of Graves' disease. This higher dose is in the range of 30 mCi, the dose at which patients are required by NRC regulations to be hospitalized. Consequently, patients with toxic functioning thyroid nodule are frequently treated with just under 30 mCi as outpatients. Treatment of an autonomous functioning nodule that does not produce enough thyroid hormone to suppress the normal thyroid tissue results in a high radiation dose to the normal thyroid tissue with a resulting high likelihood of eventual hypothyroidism. For this reason I-131 treatment should be reserved for patients in whom the nodule causes suppression of the normal thyroid tissue. These patients only uncommonly become hypothyroid following I-131 therapy.

Patients undergoing I-131 therapy for Graves' disease or autonomous functioning nodule should for 1 week avoid prolonged close contact with children or women who could be pregnant. Some authorities recommend separate eating utensils and double flushing of toilets during this period.

Although differentiated thyroid carcinoma appears to be nonfunctioning by scintigraphy when thyroid function is normal, uptake of I-131 by these tumors (but not by medullary or anaplastic carcinomas) is adequate for effective treatment if normal thyroid tissue is removed and/or ablated and if TSH levels are high. Because differentiated thyroid cancers tend to be indolent, their treatment is controversial. However, most authorities agree that I-131 therapy following surgical subtotal thyroidectomy is appropriate. Some normal thyroid tissue is always left in the thyroidal bed at surgery, partly because of the necessity of sparing parathyroid tissue. This small amount of remaining thyroid tissue usually cannot be distinguished from residual cancer scintigraphically. This situation is different from scintigraphy in patients who have a normal amount of normal thyroid tissue in that the postthyroidectomy patient has such a small amount of remaining tissue that TSH levels increase dramatically. A high TSH level stimulates differentiated thyroid cancer to increase its uptake of I-131, making tumor tissue amenable to I-131 therapy and making distant metastases visible scintigraphically. Six weeks following subtotal thyroidectomy, when TSH levels have become high, a dose of about 100 mCi of I-131 is administered to ablate the residual thyroid tissue along with residual cancer. Follow-up whole-body scintigraphy done 6 months to 1 year after successful initial I-131 therapy should show no residual uptake except for normal uptake in the nose, salivary glands, gastrointestinal tract, and urinary tract. If residual uptake suggestive of tumor is detected on this follow-up scan, a repeat dose of 100 to 200 mCi is administered (Fig. 3–7, 3–8). This process is repeated until no residual cancer is detected or until the patient's radiation burden reaches an acceptable limit, usually corresponding to a total dose of about 500 to 1000 mCi. All I-131 imaging and therapy of thyroid cancer must be carried out in the setting of high TSH levels. T4 should be discontinued about 6 weeks before imaging or therapy, and replaced with T3, which in turn is discontinued about 2 weeks before imaging or therapy.

Patients receiving I-131 therapy for thyroid cancer usually are administered doses in excess of the 30-mCi limit for outpatient treatment. Hospitalization in a room that is either shielded from or distant from other patients is necessary, as is a bathroom that is not shared. Radioactive urine is collected and shielded in the immediate posttreatment period. The patient's radiation load is measured shortly after administration of the dose of I-131 with a survey meter from a measured distance that can be repeated later.

Daily measurements are taken until this radiation load drops below the equivalent of 30 mCi, at which time discharge from the hospital is legally possible. Before discharge, contact between the patient and staff and visitors is minimized. Disposable eating utensils are used, and laundry is held in a shielded area until its radioactivity has decreased to an acceptable level. Disposable coverings can be applied to the floor and such objects as the telephone to reduce I-131 contamination. After discharge the patient should avoid prolonged, close contact with children or women who could be pregnant. Separate eating utensils should be used, toilets should be flushed twice after use, and hands should be washed carefully. These precautions should be continued for 1 week.

Potential serious complications of I-131 for thyroid cancer include malignancies, bone marrow suppression, infertility, birth defects, and anaplastic transformation of differentiated thyroid cancer. Leukemia is the malignancy that has been most convincingly associated with I-131 therapy, and only in patients who have received doses of 260 to more than 1000 mCi. The rate of occurrence is difficult to calculate because this complication is rare, but it appears to be less than 2% of all patients receiving I-131 therapy for thyroid cancer. Life-threatening marrow suppression is very unusual, especially when marrow function is carefully monitored during a series of I-131 treatments. Permanent bone marrow suppression occurs at total doses significantly greater than 200 mCi. Attempts to demonstrate an increased rate of infertility and birth defects in I-131 therapy patients and their offspring have failed. Anaplastic carcinoma occasionally develops in patients who have been treated with I-131 for differentiated thyroid carcinoma, but this phenomenon may be independent of the therapy. Radiation pneumonitis, sometimes fatal, has been reported in patients who had diffuse pulmonary metastases at the time of treatment. This phenomenon is rare and usually occurs in patients receiving high doses of I-131. Other complications include fatigue, headache, nausea, and vomiting. These effects are attributable to radiation sickness and occur in the first few days after therapy. Rare complications include pain in metastatic deposits and thyroid storm.

Parathyroid Glands

The time-tested approach to imaging **parathyroid adenomas** is dual-isotope imaging with Tc-99 pertechnetate and TL-201.

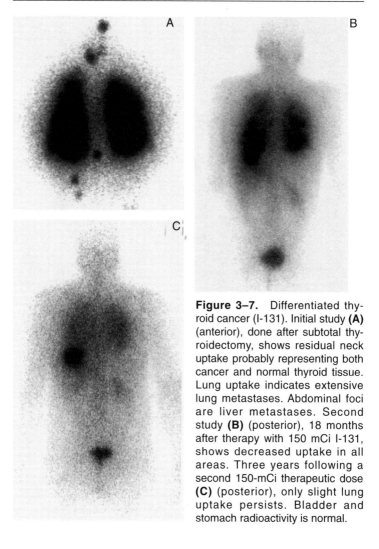

Figure 3–7. Differentiated thyroid cancer (I-131). Initial study **(A)** (anterior), done after subtotal thyroidectomy, shows residual neck uptake probably representing both cancer and normal thyroid tissue. Lung uptake indicates extensive lung metastases. Abdominal foci are liver metastases. Second study **(B)** (posterior), 18 months after therapy with 150 mCi I-131, shows decreased uptake in all areas. Three years following a second 150-mCi therapeutic dose **(C)** (posterior), only slight lung uptake persists. Bladder and stomach radioactivity is normal.

Parathyroid adenomas have an avidity for TL-201, but this tracer is also taken up by the adjacent thyroid gland. The thyroid gland shows greater uptake of Tc-99m-pertechnetate, however, and subtraction of a digital pertechnetate image from a digital TL-201 image yields an image that shows only the uptake of

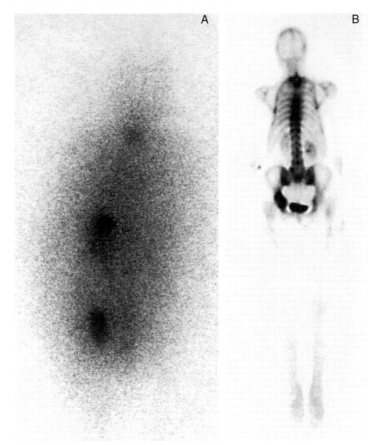

Figure 3-8. *continued*

TL-201 in the parathyroid adenoma (Fig. 3–9). Enhancement of the difference in uptake by the adenoma and normal thyroid tissue can be obtained by the administration of oral phosphates during the 3 weeks before the examination. I-123 can be substituted for Tc-99m-pectechnetate.

A newer approach uses Tc-99m-sestamibi. Following injection of tracer, images obtained at 15 minutes show uptake in both parathyroid and thyroid tissue. With time thyroid radioactivity decreases, so that at 2 hours **adenomatous or hyperplastic parathyroid** tissue shows relatively high intensity (Fig. 3–10).

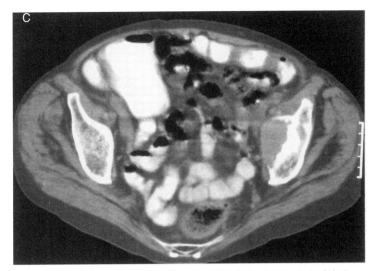

Figure 3-8. Differentiated thyroid cancer. Posterior !-131 study **(A)** done after subtotal thyroidectomy and one I-131 treatment dose shows metastatic foci at the base of the neck and in the pelvis. Gastric radioactivity is normal. A bone scan **(B)** (posterior) shows corresponding increased uptake in the upper thoracic spine and left acetabulum CT. **(C)** shows an expansile lytic and blastic left acetabular metastasis.

This may be due to greater mitochondrial density in adenomatous or hyperplastic tissue.

Adrenal Cortex

The adrenal cortex can be imaged with cholesterol or certain cholesterol derivatives because cholesterol is the precursor of adrenocortical steroids. I-131 is the usual label. Unfortunately, these radiopharmaceuticals have not been approved for general use.

I-131-19-iodocholesterol (NP-59) results in a higher target-to-background ratio than other cholesterol derivatives. The usual administered dose is 1 mCi/1.7 m^2 body surface area. Posterior images are obtained 4 to 5 days after administration. Percent uptake of the administered dose can be calculated from digital images; the normal range is 0.07 to 0.26%.

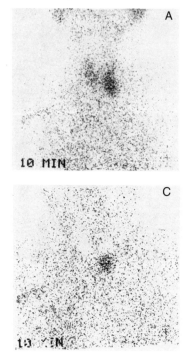

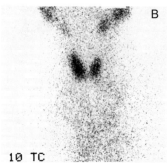

10 MIN

10 TC

1:3 MIN

Figure 3–9. Parathyroid adenoma (anterior views). T1-201 image **(A)** shows uptake in both thyroid and parathyroid tissue. T_cO_4 image **(B)** shows uptake in thyroid only. Subtracted image **(C)** shows adenoma only.

Bilateral symmetric increased uptake suggests ectopic ACTH secretion and **Cushing's syndrome.** Mildly asymmetrical uptake suggest **adrenal hyperplasia,** and unilateral uptake suggests a cortical adenoma on the side of the uptake. In case of a **cortical adenoma** causing Cushing's syndrome, ACTH production is suppressed with resultant nonvisualization of the contralateral adrenal. Bilateral nonvisualization may be caused by an **adrenal cortical carcinoma** that produces sufficient glucocorticoid to suppress pituitary ACTH but that has insufficient tracer uptake to allow visualization. The specificity of adrenal cortical scintigraphy can be increased by injecting 4 mg of dexamethasone daily for 7 days before the injection of radiotracer. Daily imaging fails to reveal normal adrenal glands through day 4; on day 5 the adrenals either are not visualized or are only faintly visualized. Cortical adenomas are seen as early (less than 5 days) unilateral uptake. Hyperplasia is seen as bilateral uptake before day 5.

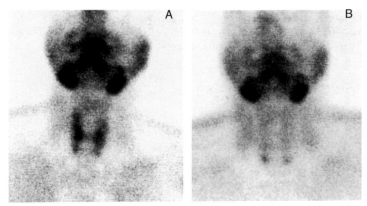

Figure 3–10. Parathyroid hyperplasia (Tc-99m-sestamibi) (anterior views). In the 15-minute image **(A)** uptake is seen in both thyroid and parathyroid tissue. The 2 hour image **(B)** shows two small foci of parathyroid hyperplasia inferior to the location of the lower poles of the thyroid.

Adrenal Medulla

I-131-methyliodobenzoguanidine (MIBG), an unapproved tracer, has been used to image the adrenal medulla. The appropriate dose is 0.5 mCi/1.7 m^2 body surface area, and thyroid uptake of free I-131 can be blocked with Lugol's solution or potassium iodine. Camera images are acquired at 24, 48, and occasionally 72 hours. The normal adrenal medulla is invisible or only faintly visualized. **Adrenal medullary hyperplasia,** sometimes seen in **multiple endocrine neoplasia type 2 syndrome,** results in bilateral increased uptake of MIBG. **Pheochromocytoma,** also seen in MEN-2 syndrome, appears as focally increased uptake at the site of either primary or metastatic tumor.

A newer tracer, In-III-octreotide, is approved for clinical use and is useful for imaging tumors of amine precursor uptake and decarboxylation (APUD) origin. This pharmaceutical shows avidity for the somatostatin receptors of **APUD tumors.** Camera images can be acquired at 4, 24, and 48 hours after injection. Target-to-background ratios are highest at 48 hours. If normal intestinal uptake interferes at 24 hours, 48-hour imaging may be helpful. Intestinal activity is usually absent at 4 hours, but target-to-background ratios may be inadequate this early. Approximate sensitivities are 86% for pheochromocytoma, 89% for neuroblastoma, 71% for medullary thyroid carcinoma, 96% for carcinoid, and 80% for pancreatic endocrine tumors.

Suggested Readings

Beierwaltes WH: The treatment of thyroid carcinoma with radioactive iodine. *Semin Nucl Med* 1978;8(1):79–94.

Culver CM, Dworkin HJ: Radiation safety considerations for post-iodine-131 thyroid cancer therapy. *J Nucl Med* 1992;33:1402–1405.

Freitas JE, Gross MD, Ripley S, Shapiro B: Radionuclide diagnosis and therapy of thyroid cancer: current status report. *Semin Nucl Med* 1985;15(2)106–131.

Krenning EP, Kwekkeboom DJ, Bakker WH, et al: somatostatin receptor scintigraphy with [^{111}In-DTPA-D-Phe^1]- and [^{123}I-Tyr^3]-octreotide: the Rotterdam experience with more than 1000 patients. *Eur J Nucl Med* 1993;20:716–731.

Nakajo M, Shapiro B, Copp J, et al: The normal and abnormal distribution of the adrenomedullary imaging agent m-[I-m-[I-131]iodobenzylguanidine (I-131 MIBG) in man: evaluation by scintigraphy. *J Nucl Med* 1983;24:672–682.

Papatheofanis FJ, Munson L: Peptide radiopharmaceutical imaging. *Appl Radiol* (June 1994):11–17.

Ramanna L, Waxman A, Braunstein G: Thallium-201 scintigraphy in differentiated thyroid cancer: comparison with radioiodine scintigraphy and serum thyroglobulin determinations. *J Nucl Med* 1991;32:441–446.

Ross DS: Evaluation of the thyroid nodule. *J Nucl Med* 1991;32:2181–2192.

Sandler MP, Patton JA: Multimodality imaging of the thyroid and parathyroids. *J Nucl Med* 1987;8:122–129.

Taillefer R, Boucher Y, Potvin C, Lambert R: detection and localization of parathyroid adenomas in patients with hyperparathyroidism using a single radionuclide imaging procedure with technetium-99m-sestamibi (doubling-phase study). *J Nucl Med* 1992;33:1801–1807.

Thrall JH, Freitas JE, Beierwaltes WH: Adrenal scintigraphy. *Semin Nucl Med* 1978;8(1):23–41.

Winzelberg GG, Hydovitz JD: Radionuclide imaging of parathyroid tumors: historical perspectives and newer techniques. *Semin Nucl Med* 1985;15(2):161–170.

Chapter 4

Esophagus, Stomach, Small Intestine, and Colon

Esophagus

Although barium studies provide excellent anatomic information about the esophagus, the radionuclide motility study provides quantitative information that is useful in the evauation of motility disorders. The patient lies supine under the gamma camera and in a single swallow ingests 10 to 15 mL of water containing 20 mCi of Tc-99m-sulfur colloid. Then dry swallows are performed every 30 seconds, and 0.5-second serial digital images are obtained. The test is terminated after several minutes, depending on monitored radioactivity remaining in the esophagus. Regions of interest are placed over the upper, middle, and lower thirds of the esophagus, and time/activity curves are generated. For each of these segments, time is measured from peak radioactivity to the point at which radioactivity has decreased to 10% of the peak value; the upper limit of normal for this time interval is 15 seconds.

Increased transit time without further distinguishing features is seen in **diabetes mellitus** and **chronic alcoholism.** In **achalasia** the prolonged transit time is often accompanied by prolonged retention of tracer in the distal third of the esophagus, although this finding is also seen in **scleroderma.** In **diffuse esophageal spasm,** imaging at the time of pain may reveal fragmentation of the tracer bolus and retrograde peristalsis.

Stomach

Gastroesophageal Reflux

Adults are studied after an overnight fast in the upright position with 0.5 to 1.0 mCi of Tc-99m-sulfur colloid dissolved in 20 to

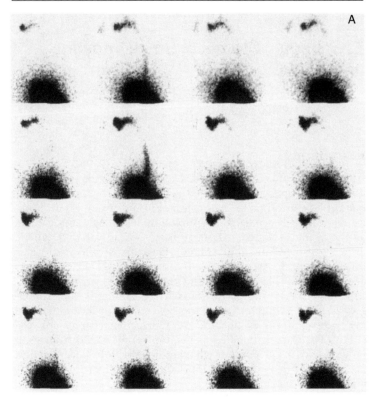

Figure 4–1. *continued*

30 mL of water followed by approximately 300 mL of water or 0.1 N hydrochloric acid in water (Fig. 4–1). Regions of interest are placed over the esophagus and stomach. Two imaging approaches have been used. In the first, 5-second images are obtained for 7 minutes. During the last two minutes the Valsalva's maneuver is performed for 10 seconds every 30 seconds. A positive study is one in which radioactivity in the esophagus is twice the magnitude of baseline. In the second approach an inflatable abdominal binder is placed and 30-second images are obtained at binder pressures of 0, 30, 60, and 90 mm Hg. This sequence is repeated after 5 minutes. A positive study is defined as greater than 1.2% of the initial gastric radioactivity appearing in the esophagus. The sensitivity of this test is in the 70 to 75%

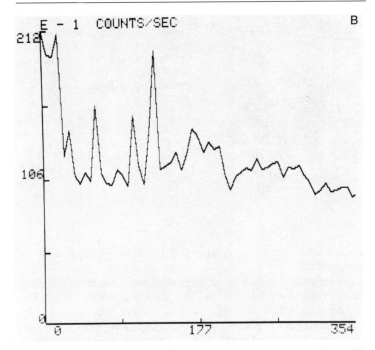

Figure 4–1. Serial 1-minute anterior images acquired over the thorax **(A)** show several episodes of gastroesophageal reflux. **(B)** Quantification from a region of interest over the esophagus shows an episode of reflux in which the peak intensity is twice the base line.

range and the specificity is about 90%. These figures are similar to those obtained with pH probe monitoring of esophageal acidity. The sensitivity of barium radiography is about 40%. Delayed (1 to 24 hours) imaging over the lungs can be used to demonstrate aspiration (Fig. 4–2).

In children, the dose of Tc-99m-sulfur colloid is reduced to 200 μCi, apple juice is used as a 30-mL diluent, and from 30 to 300 additional mL of nonradioactive apple juice is used. Continuous imaging is performed for 5 minutes. The study is considered positive when there are three or more episodes of significant elevation of the esophageal time/activity curve over baseline. The sensitivity and specificity are approximately 75 and 71%,

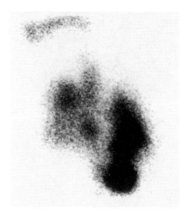

Figure 4–2. Gastric aspiration. Anterior image of chest and upper abdomen in a child with Hurler's syndrome 15 minutes after oral Tc-99m-sulfur colloid. Lung radioactivity indicates severe aspiration.

respectively. Both adults and children are studied after an overnight fast.

Gasric emptying is delayed in **gastroparesis,** the most common cause of which is diabetes mellitus, and is abnormally rapid in the **dumping syndrome.** The rate of emptying is measured by administering a radioactive meal and monitoring gastric radioactivity over time (see Fig. 4–3). The emptying rate is expresed in terms of emptying half time($t_{1/2}$). The normal range is critically dependent on several factors, including whether the meal is liquid or solid, patient positioning, patient gender, time of day of study, exercise, and physical and mental stress. Labeled solid food is a more physiologic tracer than labeled liquid. A variety of preparations has been described, including oatmeal, cream of wheat, scrambled eggs, and in vivo–labeled chicken liver. A reasonable compromise between difficulty of preparartion and stability of the label on the solid phase of the meal can be obtained by mixing 5 mCi of Tc-99m-sulfur colloid with 50 g of canned liver pâté. This mixture is then fried for 10 to 15 minutes, and about 5 g of it are mixed with 150 g of canned beef stew. The patient, having fasted overnight, is studied supine, and a region of interest is placed over the stomach. Imaging starts immediately after ingesting of the meal. Anterior and posterior acquisitions are done every 15 minutes, and count rates are calculated from the geometric mean of the anterior and posterior acquisitions (counts = [anterior count × posterior count]$^{1/2}$). For acquisitions requiring more than about 1 hour, correction should be

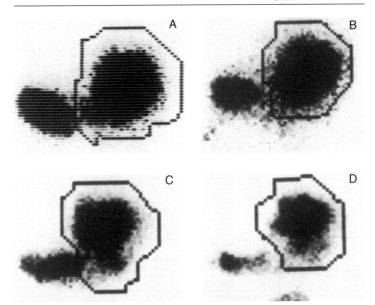

Figure 4–3. Delayed gastric emptying. The count rate within the region of interest was normalized to the immediate image **(A)**. Eighty-one percent of this level remained at 1 hour **(B)**, 55% at 2 hours **(C)**, and 42% at 3 hours **(D)**.

made for the physical half-life of Tc-99m. In normal adults, the gastric emptying half times are 92 ± 7.5 minutes in women and 60 ± 3.7 minutes in men. For liquids such as orange juice, the corresponding half emptying times are 54 ± 4.9 minutes in women and 30 ± 2.3 minutes in men. In a given normal subject, these values may vary day to day by as much as 87% for solids and 166% for liquids.

Delayed emptying of both solids and liquids is seen in **diabetes mellitus; connective-tissue disorders,** including **scleroderma;** and **Zollinger–Ellison syndrome.** Delayed emptying of only solids suggests **anorexia nervosa** or **gastritis.**

The test can be used to monitor the effect of therapeutic drugs such as metoclopramide and erythromycin on diabetic gastroparesis. These drugs have been found to have a more significant effect on the gastric emptying half times for solids than for liquids (Table 4–1).

Table 4–1.   Effects of Disease, Surgery, and Drugs on Gastric Emptying Times

	Gastric Emptying Times	
	Solids	*Liquids*
Diabetes mellitus	↑	↑
Scleroderma	↑	↑
Zollinger–Ellison	↑	↑
Anorexia nervosa	↑	—
Gastritis	↑	—
Vagotomy	—	↓
Pyloroplasty	↓	↓↓
Metaclopramide	↓↓	↓
Cisapride	↓↓	↓
Erythromycin	↓↓	↓

Small Intestine

The imaging approaches to **gastrointestinal bleeding** are angiography, labeled red blood cell (RBC) scintigraphy, and Tc-99m-sulfur colloid scintigraphy. The sulfur colloid study is the most sensitive, and angiography is the least. In sulfur colloid scintigraphy, 5 mCi of Tc-99m-sulfur colloid are administered intravenously followed immediately by imaging through 15 minutes. This test owes its sensitivity to the high contrast between the bleeding site and the nearly zero background radiation level. The approach suffers from two signifiacant disadvantages, however. First, because of the intense uptake of sulfur colloid by the liver and spleen, portions of the gastrointestinal tract near these organs cannot be evaluated accurately. Second, gastrointestinal bleeding is frequently intermittant, and sulfur colloid imaging is positive only when bleeding occurs within a few minutes of injection of the tracer. Because of these shortcomings, most institutions now use Tc-99m-RBCs.

In RBC scintigraphy, 5 mL of the patient's whole blood are removed and labeled with 20 mCi of Tc-99m. Following reinjection of the labeled cells, 1 million–count images are obtained immediately and every 10 minutes for at least 1 hour. The success of the test correlates well with the rate of bleeding. Studies are likely to be negative when bleeding rate is 0.1 mL/minute or less. At bleeding rates of about 0.15 mL/minute scintigraphy is usually weakly positive, and imaging beyond 1 hour may be necessary. For bleeding rates of 0.2 mL/min or greater, scintigraphy is weakly to strongly positive and more likely to be positive in the first hour of the study (Figs. 4–4, 4–5). Because gastrointestinal bleeding is typically intermittent, continuous imaging may be required for 24 hours or more in some patients. This can be

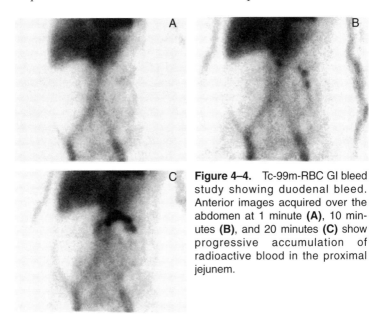

Figure 4–4. Tc-99m-RBC GI bleed study showing duodenal bleed. Anterior images acquired over the abdomen at 1 minute **(A)**, 10 minutes **(B)**, and 20 minutes **(C)** show progressive accumulation of radioactive blood in the proximal jejunem.

Figure 4–5. Tc-99m-RBC GI bleed study showing free pertechnetate and no bleed. Radioactivity concentrating in the stomach and proximal small intestine is caused by secretion of free pertechnetate in this study done with poor labeling. The large amount of excreted pertechnetate in the urinary bladder strengthens the impression of free pertechnetate rather than a gastric bleed.

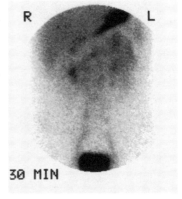

accomplished with computer control of a portable camera placed at the bedside. If the RBCs are labeled with In-111 rather than with Tc-99m, imaging can be carried out for as long as 5 days. Isolated delayed images are rarely useful unless intermittent bleeding coincidentally occurs during or shortly before the delayed image acquisition. Scintigraphic localization of the bledding site is useful in planning diagnostic or therapeutic angiography.

Meckel's diverticulum affects about 2% of the population. It occurs in the distal ileum and is therefore found typically in the right lower quadrant. About 25% of Meckel's diverticula contain gastric mucosa, which can cause adjacent ulceration because of acid secretion. However, only about 45% of Meckel's diverticula become symptomatic with bleeding, intussusception, volvulus, or diverticulitis. Most symptomatic cases appear before 2 years of age. Imaging is possible because the gastric mucosa takes up and secretes Tc-99m-pertechnetate (Fig. 4–6). The Meckel's study is performed by administering 15 mCi of Tc-99m-pertechnetate to adults or 200 μCi/kg to children intravenously. Anterior images are obtained every 5 seconds for the first minute to detect vascular lesions other than Meckel's diverticula. Static 750,000-count images are then obtained every 5 minutes for 1 hour. The bladder should be kept empty because pertechnetate is excreted by the kidneys, and a radioactive bladder can obscure an adjacent Meckel's diverticulum. The reported

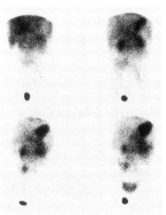

Figure 4–6. Tc-99m-TcO$_4$ Meckel's diverticulum study. Anterior images acquired over the abdomen at 1, 5, 10, and 15 minutes show progressive accumulation of tracer in a right lower quadrant Meckel's diverticulum. Accumulation of tracer in the stomach, kidneys, and urinary bladder is normal.

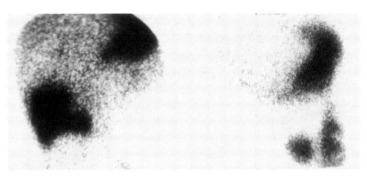

Figure 4–7. Anterior (left) and RAO (right) images from a Tc-99m-TcO$_4$ Meckel's study showing three separate right lower quadrant intestinal duplications that contain gastric mucosa.

sensitivity of the test is 50 to 85% in symptomatic patients. Higher sensitivity may be possible when 0.25 to 2.0 mg of glucagon is injected. Glucagon reduces peristalsis, thereby maintaining the focus of concentration of pertechnetate near the diverticulum and reducing contamination of the gut by gastric secretion of pertechnetate. These considerations also apply to **intestinal duplications** that contain gastric mucosa (Fig. 4–7).

The two tracers currently in common use for the evaluation of **inflammatory bowel disease** are Ga-67-citrate and In-111-labeled white blood cells (WBCs). In Ga-67 scintigraphy, 5 μCi of Ga-67 are administered, and images are obtained at 6 and 24 hours. Further images are obtained at 48 and 72 hours when necessary. Ga-67 is easily obtainable and relatively inexpensive but normally appears in the colon. For this reason interpretation may be difficult, and images on serial days are frequently necessary to distinguish normal bowel contents, which change with time, from pathologic foci, which remain anatomically constant and may become more intense relative to background over time.

In-111-WBC scintigraphy avoids the disadvantage of gallium but requires a somewhat complex labeling procedure of the patient's WBCs (Fig. 4–8). In this study, 150 to 500 μCi of In-111-labeled WBCs are injected. Early images are obtained at 3 to 6 hours and additional images at 24 or 48 hours if required. Inflammatory WBCs enter the lumen of the intestine at sites of inflammation, leading to the possibility of overestimation of the extent of bowel involvement. This phenomenon necessitates

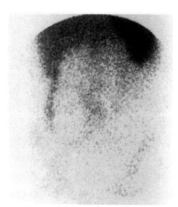

Figure 4–8. In-111-WBC study showing tracer accumulation in the ascending colon. This 24-hour abdominal image shows colonic inflammation in a 35-year-old bone marrow transplant recipient.

early images; however, late images should also be obtained if the early images are negative.

The sensitivity and specificity of In-WBC imaging are in the range of 85 to 95%. One study has shown excellent correlation between the degree of scintigraphic severity and both extent of disease and histopathologic intensity of disease in patients with **ulcerative colitis** or **Crohn's disease.** The study has proved useful in monitoring the result of therapy; however, multiple studies should be considered with caution because of the high radiation dose to the spleen.

Ischemic enterocolitis has been reported as a cause of increased uptake of In-111-WBCs, presumably because of the inflammation associated with the ischemia. Necrotizing enterocolitis of the newborn can be studied eith Tc-99m-pyrophosphate (PYP). Three hundred thousand-count images are obtained 2 hours after injection of 500 µCi of Tc-99m-PYP. Increased abdominal uptake, either diffuse or focal, of PYP, occurs in necrotizing enterocolitis with a sensitivity of about 80%.

Protein-losing enteropathy can be confirmed with the intravenous administration of Tc-99m-HSA. After an administered dose of 20 mCi, small intestine activity is seen at 30 minutes and colonic activity at 24 hours in positive studies.

Colon

Quantitative measurement of colonic transit is occasionally valuable in the evaluation and treatment of patients with severe constipation. Orally administered tracers that have been studied for this application include I-131-cellulose and In-111-DTPA. Of these two tracers, In-111-DTPA is more easily obtainable and appears to yield studies that are just as valid as those done with I-131-cellulose. Following an overnight fast, 1.0 mCi of In-111-DTPA are administered with a small meal. Computer-generated geometric mean images are reconstructed from anterior and posterior acquisitions done at 6, 24, 48, 72, and 96 hours. Total abdominal radioactivity at 6 hours is taken as 100%. In normal subjects retained radioactivity within a colonic region of interest is about 12% at 48 hours as compared with about 80% in constipated patients. If desired, segmental retention can be calculated to localize pathology.

Suggested Readings

Blumhagen JD, Rudd TG, Christie DL: Gastroesophageal reflux in children: radionuclide gastroesophography. *AJR* 1980;135:1001–1004.

Caride VJ, Touloukian RJ, Ablow RC, Lange RC, Matthews T: Abdominal and hepatic uptake of ^{99m}Tc-pyrophosphate in neonatal necrotizing enterocolitis. *Radiology* 1981;139:205–209.

Channer KS, Virgee JP: Oesophageal function tests: are they of value? *Clin Radiol* 1985;36:493–496.

Datz FL, Christian PE, Hutson WR, Moore JG, Morton KA: Physiological and pharmacological interventions in radionuclide imaging of the tubular gastrointestinal tract. *Semin Nucl Med* 1991;21(2):140–152.

Datz FL, Christian PE, Moore J: Gender-related differences in gastric emptying. *J Nucl Med* 1987;28:1204–1207.

Davies ER: Radionuclides and the gut. *Clin Radiol* 1990;42:80–84. Review.

Ferrant A, Dehasque N, Leners N, Meunier H: Scintigraphy with In-111-labeled red cells in intermittent gastrointestinal bleeding. *J Nucl Med* 1980;21:844–845.

Murphy PH: Acceptance test and quality control of gamma cameras, including SPECT. *J Nucl Med* 1987;28:1221–1227.

Rothstein RD, Alavi A: The role of scintigraphy in the management of inflammatory bowel disease. *J Nucl Med* 1991;32:856–859.

Rowe CC, Berkovic SF, Austin MC, et al.: Visual and quantitative analysis of interictal SPECT with technetium-99m-HMPAO in temporal lobe epilepsy. *J Nucl Med* 199;32:1688–1694.

Smart RC, McLean RG, Gaston-Parry D, Barbagallo S, et al.: Comparison of oral iodine-131-cellulose and indium-111-DTPA as tracers for colon transit scintigraphy: analysis by colon activity profiles. *J Nucl Med* 1991;32:1668–1674.

Smith R, Copely DJ, Bolen FH: ^{99m}Tc-RBC scintigraphy: correlation of gastrointestinal bleeding rates with scintigraphic findings. *AJR* 1987;148:869–874.

Styles CB, Holt S, Bowes KL, Jewell L, Hooper HR: Gastroesophageal reflux and transit scintigraphy: a comparison with esophageal biopsy in patients with heartburn. *J Canad Assoc Radiol* 1984;35:124–127.

Thrall JH, Swanson DP: Diagnostic interventions in nuclear medicine. *Curr Probl Diagn Radiol* 1989;18(1):1–37.

Velasco N, Pope CE II, Gannan RM, Roberts P, Hill LD: Measurement of esophageal reflux by scintigraphy. *Dig Dis Sci* 1984;29:977–982.

Chapter 5

Liver, Biliary Tract, Spleen, and Pancreas

Liver

The liver parenchyma contains systems of two main cell types, the hepatocytes and the Kupffer cells. The hepatocytes perform the liver's metabolic functions such as bile production, and the Kupffer cells are histiocytic cells of the reticuloendothelial system. Current hepatocyte imaging is done with Tc-99m-diisopropyl-IDA (Tc-99m-DISIDA) or similar agents. The examination is tailored to the clinical problem, but generally 5 mCi of Tc-99m-DISIDA are administered, and anterior images are obtained at 5, 10, 15, 30, 45, and 60 minutes. The acquisition time and photographic parameters are held constant so that changes in intensity can be evaluated. Acquisition time is such that when the liver is maximally intense (about 15 minutes after injection in normal subjects) 500,000 counts are acquired. Oblique views and delayed images are obtained as necessary (Fig. 5–1).

Kupffer cell imaging is done with 6 mCi of Tc-99m-sulfur colloid (Tc-99m-SC) followed by anterior and posterior imaging at 20 minutes after injection. Oblique and lateral views are added as necessary; 500,000-count images are acquired.

Focal Lesions

Metastases are the commonest liver **tumors** and are generally best evaluated with computed tomography and ultrasound because of the excellent spatial resolution of these modalities, and because structures outside of the liver can also be evaluated. Several primary liver tumors have distinct scintigraphic appearances, and for these lesions scintigraphy can be helpful. In particular, malignant tumors do not contain Kupffer cells, so Tc-99m-SC uptake in a tumor excludes the possibility of malignancy.

Focal nodular hyperplasia is a benign tumor that occurs typi-

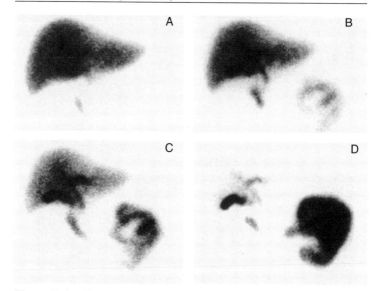

Figure 5–1. Normal Tc-99m-DISIDA study. Anterior views at 5 minutes **(A)**, 15 minutes **(B)**, 30 minutes **(C)**, and 60 minutes **(D)**. Parenchymal intensity should peak by 15 minutes or earlier, as is the case here. Intrahepatic bile ducts should be maximally intense at 45 minutes or earlier (approximately 30 minutes in this case). Parenchymal radioactivity should decrease to less than one-third of its peak intensity by 1 hour. Tracer should be seen in either the gallbladder or intestine by 15 minutes or earlier. (The intestine is seen at 5 minutes in this case.) The gallbladder should be visualized at 60 minutes or earlier (15 minutes in this case). Additional images are often obtained at 10 and 45 minutes. Right lateral and right anterior oblique views are obtained as needed.

cally in young women; it may be more common in women using oral contraceptives. This lesion frequently contains both Kupffer cells and hepatocytes, and usually shows normal or increased uptake of both Tc-99m-SC and Tc-99m-DISIDA (Fig. 5–2).

Hepatic adenoma consists of benign hepatocyte-derived cells. Whether adenomas contain Kupffer cells is controversial. Some studies claim they do not, and some claim that all adenomas contain Kupffer cells. However, all reports indicate that most (77 to 100%) hepatic adenomas do not show Tc-99m-SC uptake. The relatively well-differentiated hepatocytes are capable of extracting Tc-99m-DISIDA from the blood, but the lack of

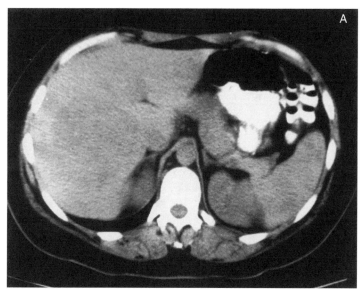

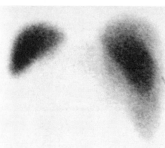

Figure 5–2. Focal nodular hyperplasia. Computed tomography **(A)** shows a large low-density lesion in the posterior aspect of the right hepatic lobe. Posterior Tc-99m-sulfur colloid image **(B)** shows increased uptake in the region of the tumor, indicating the presence of Kupffer cells and therefore excluding a malignant tumor.

bile ducts prevents excretion of this tracer. The typical scintigraphic appearance of hepatic adenoma, then, is no uptake on Tc-99m-SC scintigraphy, and gradually increasing relative intensity on Tc-99m-DISIDA imaging with retention of tracer in the tumor as surrounding normal parenchyma loses radioactivity (Fig. 5–3). The distinction of hepatic adenoma from other benign lesions is important because adenomas are prone to hemorrhage and infarction, and because a small percentage of adenomas undergo malignant change.

Regenerating nodules occur in cirrhotic livers and contain

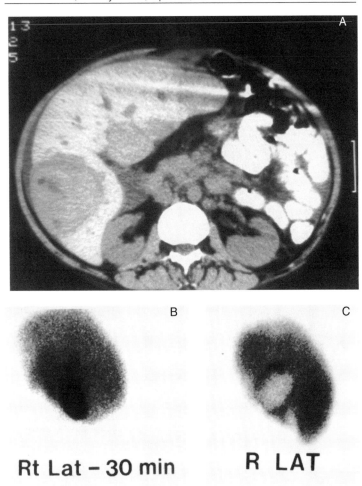

Rt Lat – 30 min   **R LAT**

Figure 5–3. Hepatic adenomas. Computed tomography **(A)** shows a low-density tumor in the right lobe and another in the caudate lobe of the liver. Right lateral scintigraphic image done with Tc-99m-DISIDA **(B)** shows increased uptake in the region of the right lobe mass adjacent to the gallbladder, indicating the presence of functioning hepatocytes in the tumor. Tc-99m-sulfur colloid imaging **(C)** shows decreased uptake in the tumor, reflecting the absence of Kupffer cells; a rim of increased uptake around the tumor is probably the result of hyperemia.

both Kupffer cells and hepatocytes. These lesions usually show normal uptake of both Tc-99m-SC and Tc-99m-DISIDA.

Fatty infiltration of the liver may be focal and can be detected by computed tomography or ultrasound. The fat infiltration does not affect Kupffer cell or hepatocyte function, so Tc-99m-SC and Tc-99m-DISIDA imaging are both normal.

Cavernous hemangioma is a vascular lesion that contains neither hepatocytes nor Kupffer cells. This lesion always appears photon deficient on Tc-99m-SC and Tc-99m-DISIDA imaging. Because cavernous hemangiomas usually have high blood volume but low blood flow, perfusion studies done with nondiffusible tracers such as Tc-99m-RBCs show photon deficiency in the region of the tumor in early images (first minute) but increased radioactivity on delayed images (greater than one-half hour) (Figs. 5–4, 5–5). The more important of these two criteria is the second, although increased tracer in delayed images may occur in hypervascular tumors other than hemangioma, such as some hepatomas and hemangiosarcomas. These tumors, however, typically show increased rather than decreased perfusion on early rapid-sequence images, and for this reason the early images are important in the diagnosis of hemangioma. When single photon emission computed tomography (SPECT) imaging is used, the sensitivity of the test in a population of patients with hemangiomas ranging in size from 1 to 5 cm is 74%. For tumors greater than 2 cm in diameter, the sensitivity is 88%, and for tumors between 4 and 5 cm in diameter it is nearly 100%. Specificity is in the range of 90 to 100%. The noninvasive diagnosis of hemangioma is important because this tumor is common, occurring in up to 7% of autopsies.

Hepatomas contain no Kupffer cells, and the hepatocyte-derived tumor cells are variably differentiated. As a result, hepatomas are photon-deficient in Tc-99m-SC imaging. Most hepatomas are not well enough differentiated to show significant uptake of Tc-99m-DISIDA within the first half hour after injection, but they may show uptake on delayed images. At least 95% of hepatomas show uptake of Ga-67 that is equal to or greater than the surrounding liver (Fig. 5–6).

Lacerations with hematomas show no uptake of Tc-99m-SC. Early (less than 10 minutes) Tc-99m-DISIDA images show no uptake. However, if the hematoma communicates with the bile ducts, tracer may eventually appear within the laceration (Fig.

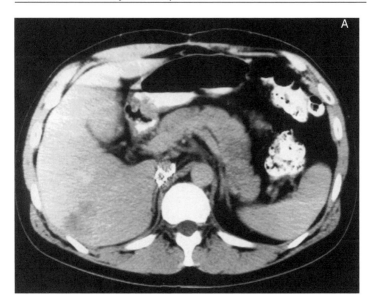

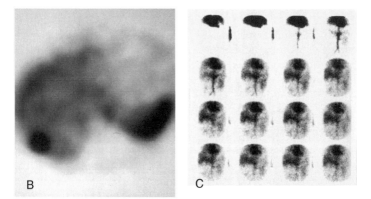

Figure 5–4. Cavernous hemangioma. Computed tomography **(A)** shows a low-density mass in the posterior aspect of the right lobe of the liver. A 1-hour transaxial SPECT image **(B)** at the level of the lesion shows increased uptake, indicating high blood volume in the lesion. Anterior 2-second perfusion images **(C)** fail to show the increased perfusion often seen in malignant tumors but uncommonly seen in cavernous hemangiomas.

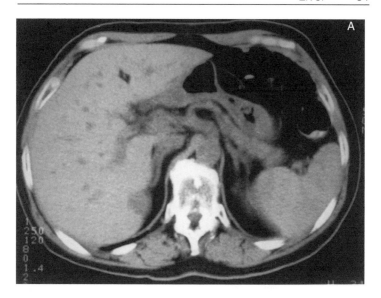

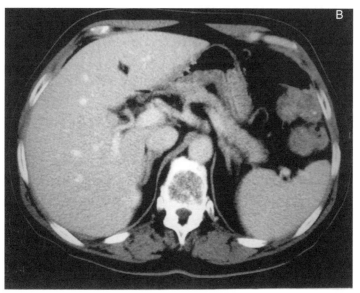

Figure 5–5. *continued*

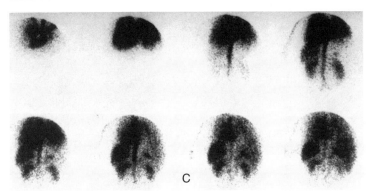

C

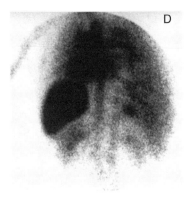

D

Figure 5–5. Hepatic metastases. Computed tomography—**(A)** without contrast, **(B)** with contrast—shows a small enhancing mass in the posteromedial aspect of the right lobe. Posterior scintigraphic perfusion **(C)** and immediate blood pool **(D)** images show tracer activity in this lesion, a finding commonly seen in metastases but rarely seen in cavernous hemangiomas. Transaxial SPECT images **(E)** show minimally increased tracer in the lesion relative to surrounding liver; this finding is somewhat suggestive of cavernous hemangioma, but, as in this case, can be seen in malignant tumors.

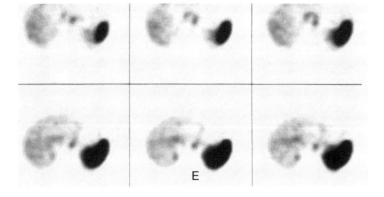

E

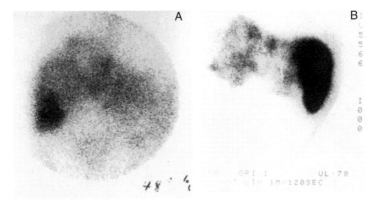

Figure 5–6. Hepatoma. A 48-hour anterior gallium-67 image **(A)** shows increased uptake in the inferior aspect of the right lobe of the liver. An anterior Tc-99m-sulfur colloid image **(B)** shows decreased, inhomogeneous uptake in the liver, with no uptake in the inferior aspect of the right lobe. These findings are suggestive of hepatoma in a cirrhotic liver. The spleen is enlarged and shows increased uptake of Tc-99m-sulfur colloid, the result of liver failure and portal hypertension.

ducts, tracer may eventually appear within the laceration (Fig. 5–7).

Abscesses (Fig. 5–8) behave similarly to lacerations except that Tc-99m-SC imaging occasionally shows a rim of increased uptake around the photon-deficient abscess, possibly resulting from increased perfusion of tissue around the abscess. Demonstration of communication of an abscess cavity with the bile ducts may be useful in treatment planning. Such communication provides a drainage path for the abscess; critically ill patients may avoid surgical drainage when such a communication is demonstrated.

Diffuse Parenchymal Disease

Most diseases of the liver parenchyma affect both the Kupffer cells and the hepatocytes. Tc-99m-sulfur colloid uptake is therefore decreased in diseases that affect liver function, even though the Kupffer cells are not the metabolically active cells of the liver. This effect is manifested by a decrease in liver uptake relative to uptake in the spleen and marrow and is sometimes referred to as colloid shift (Fig. 5–9). In a posterior image that is properly

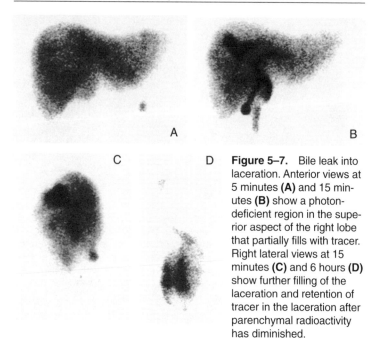

Figure 5–7. Bile leak into laceration. Anterior views at 5 minutes **(A)** and 15 minutes **(B)** show a photon-deficient region in the superior aspect of the right lobe that partially fills with tracer. Right lateral views at 15 minutes **(C)** and 6 hours **(D)** show further filling of the laceration and retention of tracer in the laceration after parenchymal radioactivity has diminished.

exposed for the liver in a patient with diffuse liver disease, Tc-99m-sulfur colloid imaging shows skeletal structures clearly because of the increased marrow uptake. These structures are not ordinarily seen well in a properly exposed image of a normal liver. Marrow uptake of Tc-99m-micro albumin colloid, another Kupffer cell imaging agent, is roughly twice that of Tc-99m-SC. As a result, the bones may be faintly seen in the posterior view of a normal liver imaged with this agent.

Parenchymal diseases that affect liver function may be conceptually categorized as (1) affecting primarily the hepatocytes or (2) causing decreased bile flow in the face of normal hepatocyte function (intrahepatic cholestasis). This distinction can be made effectively with Tc-99m-DISIDA imaging. A second distinction can be made between intrahepatic cholestasis and surgically amenable large-bile-duct mechanical obstruction.

Causes of **hepatocyte dysfunction** include hepatitis of multiple etiologies, cirrhosis, long-standing biliary obstruction, and effects of drugs. The major finding of hepatocyte dysfunction in Tc-

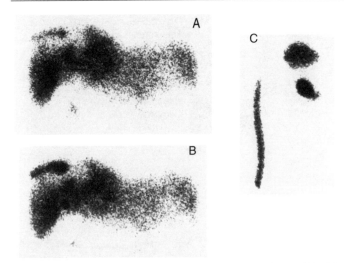

Figure 5–8. Amebic abscess. Anterior views at 5 minutes **(A)**, 15 minutes **(B)**, and 4 hours **(C)** show progressive accumulation of tracer in a photon-deficient abscess in the superior aspect of the right lobe. A drain extends from the abscess and down the right side of the patient.

99m-DISIDA imaging is a decrease in the amplitude of the peak of the parenchymal time–activity curve; a secondary lesser effect is a delay in the time of the peak. Images obtained around the time of the peak (the 10-or 15 minute images), when properly exposed, show distinct cardiac blood pool radioactivity when the hepatocytes are dysfunctional. When hepatocyte dysfunction is severe, cardiac blood pool radioactivity intensity may exceed the peak hepatic parenchymal radioactivity intensity (Fig. 5–10).

Intrahepatic cholestasis occurs when bile excretion is impaired diffusely throughout the liver. There may be concomitant hepatocyte dysfunction. Causes of intrahepatic cholestasis include viral and alcoholic hepatitis; drugs, including steroids; gram-negative infection; total parenteral nutrition; primary biliary cirrhosis; ascending cholangitis; and intrahepatic biliary hypoplasia. The main effect of intrahepatic cholestasis on imaging is to decrease the rate at which the hepatic parenchymal intensity drops following its peak. In cases of intrahepatic cholestasis with normal hepatocyte function, the 10- and 15-minute images show normal parenchymal intensity and little or no discernible cardiac blood

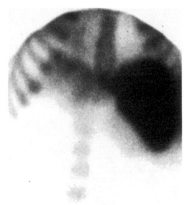

Figure 5–9. End-stage cirrhosis. This anterior Tc-99m-sulfur colloid image shows decreased inhomogeneous uptake in a shrunken liver in the right upper quadrant. The relative intensity of the enlarged spleen and of the marrow is increased ("colloid shift").

pool radioactivity (Fig. 5–11). Subsequent images show abnormally slow decrease in parenchymal intensity, and appearance of tracer in the biliary tree and small intestine may be delayed.

Ascites resulting from liver disease is sometimes treated with indwelling peritoneal to venous shunt valves. The function of these shunts can be tested by injecting 1 to 5 mCi of Tc-99m-macroaggregated albumin into the ascites fluid and then imaging

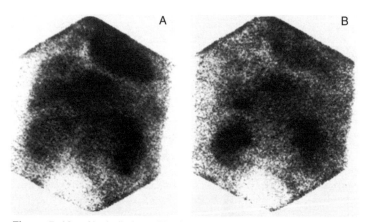

Figure 5–10. Alcoholic hepatitis. Anterior views at 5 minutes **(A)** and 45 minutes **(B)** show much greater than the expected level of radioactivity in the cardiac blood pool and other structures relative to hepatic radioactivity, indicating severe hepatocyte dysfunction.

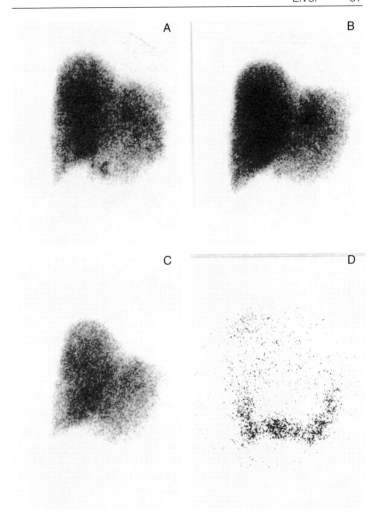

Figure 5–11. Intrahepatic cholestasis. Anterior views at 5 minutes **(A)**, 60 minutes **(B)**, 3 hours **(C)**, and 24 hours **(D)**. Absence of visible cardiac blood pool radioactivity at 5 minutes indicates normal hepatocyte uptake function. Parenchymal intensity decreases abnormally slowly, and tracer is not seen outside the liver until 24 hours. These findings suggest biliary obstruction. Failure of this study to demonstrate a point of obstruction in a large bile duct suggests diffuse obstruction, in this case intrahepatic cholestasis associated with primary biliary cirrhosis.

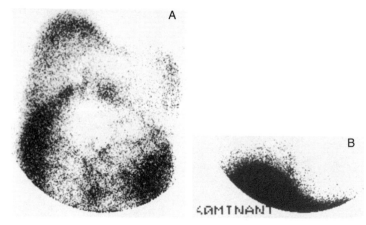

Figure 5–12. Nonfunctioning peritoneal to venous shunt. Anterior views were done at 10 minutes over the abdomen **(A)** and at 1 hour over the chest **(B).** These images were obtained following an injection of Tc-99m-MAA into the ascites fluid. Failure of tracer to move from the peritoneum to the shunt into the systemic venous circulation and then into the lungs indicates failure of the shunt device.

over the lungs for 1 hour. When the shunt is functioning, tracer shifts from the abdomen to the lungs (Fig. 5–12).

Biliary Tract

Findings that suggest **biliary obstruction** on Tc-99m-DISIDA imaging include inappropriately slow decrease in parenchymal radioactivity (as in intrahepatic cholestasis), delayed appearance of radioactive bile outside the liver (greater than 15 minutes), delay of the time of peak intrahepatic bile duct radioactivity to greater than 45 minutes, and appearance of a change in the caliber or intensity of a bile duct at the point of obstruction (Figs. 5–13, 5–14). Not all these signs may be present in extrahepatic obstruction, and bile duct dilation alone may not be associated with obstruction (Fig. 5–15). If the obstruction is complete, the criteria that involve the appearance of the bile ducts cannot be used, because the ducts and gallbladder are rarely visualized in complete biliary obstruction; the reason for this situation is that imaging usually takes place long enough after the obstruction has occurred that bile flow has stopped completely.

The effect of extrahepatic biliary obstruction on the parenchymal time–activity curve is the same as that in intrahepatic cholestasis: the rate of descent of the curve following its peak is decreased. When the obstruction has not been present long enough to cause secondary hepatocyte damage, the 5- and 10-minute images show a normal hepatic to cardiac intensity ratio (cardiac blood pool invisible or nearly invisible), but hepatocyte function and therefore tracer uptake decline over the days to weeks following the onset of obstruction.

Distinguishing between **extrahepatic biliary atresia** and **neonatal hepatitis**—common causes of neonatal jaundice that occur with roughly equal frequency—is important because biliary atresia is amenable to surgery. Of the types of congenital biliary hypoplasia and biliary atresia, types in which the intrahepatic bile ducts are relatively normal and the extrahepatic ducts are completely obstructed by one or more atretic segments are by far the most common. The hepatocytes are not significantly damaged by the obstruction during the first 2 months or so of life. This situation is thus a special case of complete extrahepatic biliary obstruction with normal hepatocyte function. Tc-99m-DISIDA imaging in such patients shows normal hepatocyte intensity relative to the cardiac blood pool at 10 minutes, no significant drop in parenchymal intensity with time beyond 10 minutes (except for physical decay of the Tc-99m label), and no appearance of radioactive bile outside the liver through 24 hours (Fig. 5–16). These findings are in contrast to those of neonatal

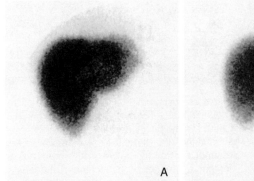
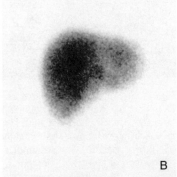

A   B

Figure 5–13.   *continued*

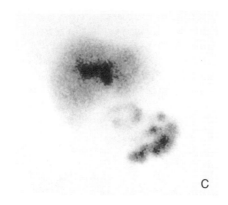

C

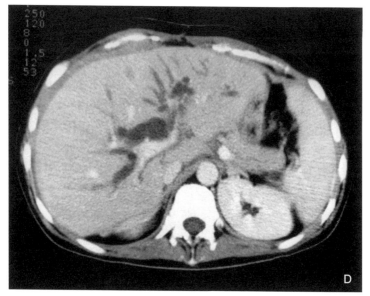

D

Figure 5–13. Common bile duct obstruction. Anterior Tc-99m-DISIDA images at 5 minutes **(A),** 1 hour **(B),** and 4 hours **(C)** show normal hepatocyte uptake function but abnormally slow decrease of parenchymal radioactivity. An abrupt change in the intensity of the common bile duct at the porta hepatis with proximal dilation indicates partial mechanical obstruction at this point. Computed tomography **(D)** confirms intrahepatic biliary dilation, in this case secondary to gastric carcinoma metastases in the porta hepatis.

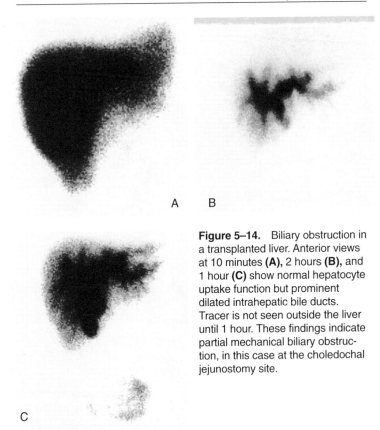

Figure 5–14. Biliary obstruction in a transplanted liver. Anterior views at 10 minutes **(A)**, 2 hours **(B)**, and 1 hour **(C)** show normal hepatocyte uptake function but prominent dilated intrahepatic bile ducts. Tracer is not seen outside the liver until 1 hour. These findings indicate partial mechanical biliary obstruction, in this case at the choledochal jejunostomy site.

hepatitis in which the hepatocytes are significantly damaged and in which there is frequently a concomitant element of intrahepatic cholestasis. In neonatal hepatitis, Tc-99m-DISIDA imaging typically shows decreased parenchymal intensity at 10 minutes relative to the cardiac blood pool, and radioactive bile outside the liver is seen by 24 hours (Fig. 5–17). The distinction between these two conditions is less clear-cut if imaging occurs late enough in life (greater than 2 months of age) when the hepatocytes become significantly damaged or in cases of neonatal hepatitis in which bile production is so poor that extrahepatic radioactive bile is never seen; these cases must be classified as

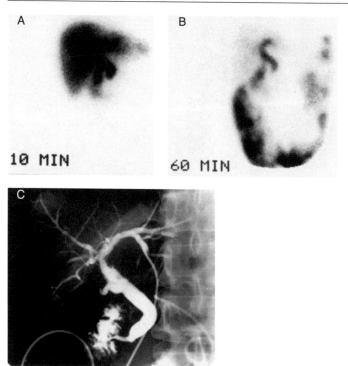

Figure 5–15. Anterior Tc-99m-DISIDA images (**A**, 10 minutes; **B**, 60 minutes) show normal hepatocyte function and a common bile duct that is prominent but that shows rapidly decreasing intensity. The parenchymal intensity also decreases appropriately, and these findings suggest that the dilation is not associated with current obstruction. Contrast injection of a biliary stent (**C**) shows biliary dilation secondary to previous obstruction but free flow of contrast through the biliary tree. The stent traverses a biliary carcinoma.

indeterminate. The accuracy of Tc-99m-DISIDA imaging in neonatal hepatitis and biliary atresia may be improved by pretreatment with phenobarbital, which increases the uptake and excretion of Tc-99m-DISIDA. Patients are administered 2.5 mg/kg twice daily for at least 5 days before the injection of 50 <gm>Ci/kg of Tc-99m-DISIDA. The accuracy of the test is greater than 90%.

Tc-99m-DISIDA imaging is very effective in the detection of

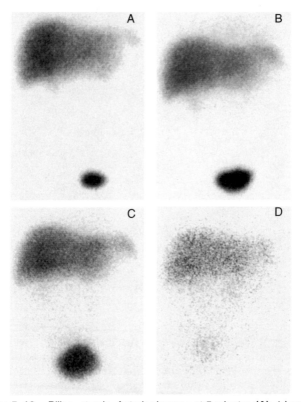

Figure 5–16.   Biliary atresia. Anterior images at 5 minutes **(A)**, 1 hour **(B)**, 4 hours **(C)**, and 24 hours **(D)** show normal hepatocyte function but abnormally slow decrease in parenchymal intensity. Biliary or intestinal tracer is never seen outside the liver. These findings indicate high-grade biliary obstruction of indeterminant location; in this case the cause was extrahepatic biliary atresia.

bile leaks because of the inherently high contrast of this study compared with roentgenographic procedures. In general, leaks appear as collections of radioactivity that enlarge and increase in intensity with time but that do not conform to the expected location and shape of the biliary tree, small intestine, or colon (Fig. 5–18). Leaks may be within the liver, as in abscesses (Fig. 5–8) and lacerations (Fig. 5–7), or outside the liver, as in anastomotic leaks, gallbladder rupture, and penetrating trauma.

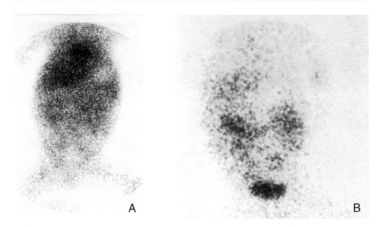

A   B

Figure 5–17. Neonatal hepatitis. Anterior views at 5 minutes **(A)** and at 24 hours **(B)** show decreased hepatocyte function as indicated by high levels of persistent tracer in the cardiac blood pool and other extrahepatic structures at 5 minutes but presence of tracer in the colon at 24 hours. These findings indicate severe hepatocyte dysfunction but without complete obstruction.

Shortly after the introduction of IDA derivatives such as Tc-99m-DISIDA, the discovery was made that imaging with these tracers could provide an extremely accurate test for **acute cholecystitis** (Fig. 5–19). Following administration injection of tracer to a patient with an otherwise normal hepatobiliary system and with appropriate dietary preparation, the normal gallbladder is visualized within 1 hour, and the acutely inflamed gallbladder is not visualized through 4 hours. A frequent finding in patients with acute cholecystitis is a rim of increased tracer uptake in the hepatic parenchyma adjacent to the gallbladder (Fig. 5–20). This finding is only infrequently encountered when acute cholecystitis is absent. Thus if the rim is seen at 1 hour, acute cholecystitis is likely. Visualization may occur between 1 and 4 hours in patients with chronic cholecystitis. The dietary preparation is appropriate when the patient has eaten 2 to 12 hours before the study. Prolonged fasting may result in a false-positive result (nonvisualization of the gallbladder). After a prolonged fast, the gallbladder is maximally expanded, and the rate of water transport across its mucosa is minimal; these two factors prevent the flow of bile into the gallbladder. If food is ingested less than 2 hours before the test, this may also result in a false-positive

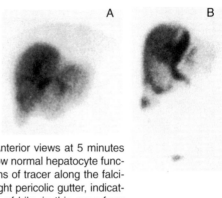

Figure 5–18. Bile leak. Anterior views at 5 minutes **(A)** and 60 minutes **(B)** show normal hepatocyte function but abnormal collections of tracer along the falciform ligament and in the right pericolic gutter, indicating intraperitoneal leakage of bile, in this case from the choledochojejunostomy in a transplanted liver.

result, although patients with acute cholecystitis are unlikely to have eaten recently. There are two approaches to the problem of the prolonged fast. The first and more physiologic is the administration of cholecystokinin (CCK) or sincalide, the C-terminal octapeptide of CCK. Sincalide is more easily available and effectively induces gallbladder contraction. To reduce the likelihood of a false-positive Tc-99m-DISIDA gallbladder study for acute cholecystitis, 0.02 mg/kg of CCK is given 30 minutes before tracer injection. The gallbladder contracts almost immediately, and by the time imaging starts, the gallbladder is expanding, allowing entry of bile into the gallbladder.

The second approach to the scintigraphic diagnosis of acute cholecystitis in the patient who has fasted for longer than 12 hours involves the use of morphine. Intravenous injection of 0.04 mg/kg of morphine causes contraction of the sphincter of Oddi, with resulting increase in the biliary tract pressure. This increase in pressure is usually adequate to force some radioactive bile into a gallbladder that is not acutely inflamed. The morphine can be injected immediately before tracer is injected, but then the diagnosis of chronic cholecystitis is impossible, a sacrifice that may be of little importance in the case of suspected acute cholecystitis. Alternatively, the morphine can be injected at 30 to 60 minutes after tracer injection if the gallbladder is not yet visualized by this time. Delaying morphine injection for up to 30 minutes will save some patients the morphine injection because by this time the gallbladder may be visualized; however,

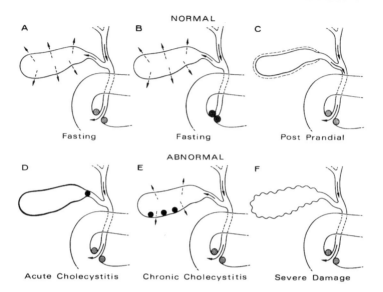

Figure 5–19. Visualization of the gallbladder depends on the direction of bile flow in the cystic duct. **(A)** In the normal fasting subject, bile flowing from the liver divides at the cystic duct. Because the gallbladder wall absorbs water and because the gallbladder may be expanding, some bile flow into the cystic duct; if Oddi's sphincter is relaxed, some bile flows into the common bile duct and duodenum. **(B)** In some normal subjects, Oddi's sphincter is closed, resulting in delayed visualization of the duodenum. **(C)** In the normal postprandial subject, contraction of gallbladder reverses bile flow in the cystic duct; tracer does not enter the gallbladder. **(D)** In acute cholecystitis, the cystic duct is obstructed by a stone or edema or both; bile does not enter the gallbladder. **(E)** In chronic cholecystitis, water absorption by the damaged gallbladder wall may be slowed, resulting in delayed visualization of the gallbladder. **(F)** If chronic inflammation or a tumor has severely damaged the gallbladder wall, water absorption may be absent and the gallbladder volume may be fixed. The gallbladder is not visualized by 24 hours.

the diagnosis of chronic cholecystitis will still be impossible. Administering morphine at 60 minutes after tracer injection when the gallbladder has not yet been visualized allows for the diagnosis of either chronic or acute cholecystitis. The disadvantage of this method is that by 60 minutes insufficient tracer excretion may remain for reliable gallbladder visualization, necessitating a second injection of Tc-99m-DISIDA. When morphine is used the gallbladder should be visualized by 1.5 hours

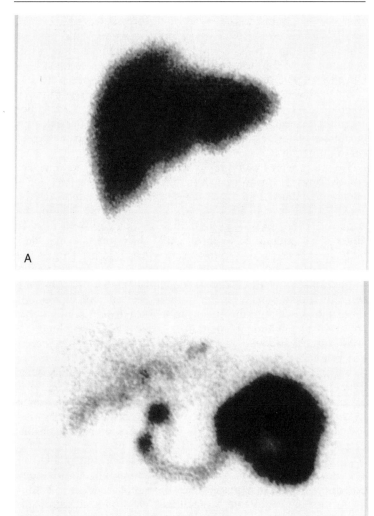

Figure 5–20. Acute cholecystitis. Anterior images were done at 5 minutes **(A)** and 60 minutes **(B).** Hepatocyte function is normal, and there is no evidence for biliary obstruction. The gallbladder is not seen and was not seen on delayed images. Increased residual tracer in the hepatic parenchyma adjacent to the gallbladder fossa (rim sign) is highly suggestive of acute cholecystitis.

after tracer administration; if it is not, acute cholecystitis is indicated. Morphine is frequently administered with the goal of reducing the duration of the test from a maximum of 4 hours to a maximum of 1.5 hours rather than to compensate for a prolonged fast. The overall sensitivity of the test is between 95 and 100%, and the specificity is between 80 and 100% regardless of whether a 4-hour image, sincalide, or morphine is used. However, excessive false-positive results have been reported with morphine in severely ill patients, especially those on total parenteral nutrition.

The accuracy of scintigraphy in the diagnosis of acute cholecystitis depends on normal liver function and bile excretion. If uptake is abnormal and especially if bile flow is reduced to the extent that the small intestine is not visualized by 1 hour, the accuracy of the test is reduced. In these cases imaging through 24 hours in an attempt to establish gallbladder function may partially restore some of the test accuracy lost as a result of the impaired hepatobiliary function. In a few percent of patients with acute cholecystitis, especially severely ill hospitalized patients, the cystic duct may remain patent. In these cases of acute acalculous cholecystitis, scintigraphy may be falsely negative. A scintigraphic approach to this urgent situation is the In-111 white blood cell (WBC) study, although imaging through 24 hours may be necessary to establish a diagnosis of acute cholecystitis.

The vast majority (95%) of patients with **chronic cholecystitis** have gallstones. The diagnosis of gallstones by ultrasound is extremely accurate, and scintigraphy is ordinarily not indicated in these patients. However, the 5% of chronic cholecystitis patients who do not have stones may have abdominal pain but ultrasonically normal gallbladders. Diagnosis of acalculous chronic cholecystitis can be made by measuring the gallbladder ejection fraction with Tc-99m-DISIDA scintigraphy. In this study a region of interest is placed over the gallbladder on a 1-hour image and the count rate is measured. Then 0.02 mg/kg of sincalide is administered over 3 minutes. An image is then obtained at 45 minutes and for the same acquisition time as was required to obtain a 500,000-count image before sincalide administration. Regions of interest are placed over the gallbladder or the pre- and postsincalide images. The gallbladder ejection fraction is calculated by subtracting the background-corrected postsincalide count rate from the background-corrected presincalide count rate and dividing the result by the background-corrected presincalide

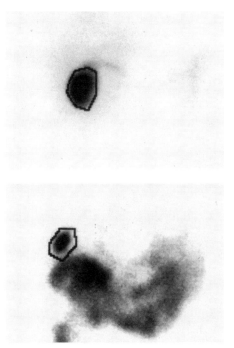

Figure 5–21. Gallbladder ejection fraction determination. Regions of interest placed over the gallbladder before and after the administration of cholecystokinin are used to measure gallbladder radioactivity from which the ejection fraction is calculated. In this case the ejection fraction was normal.

count rate (Fig. 5–21). An ejection fraction below 35% is abnormal and suggestive of chronic cholecystitis.

Spleen

The tracers used in splenic imaging can be classified as colloidal or noncolloidal. Colloids contain insoluble particles that remain in suspension and are phagocytized by the reticuloendothelial system (RES) when given intravenously. The marrow, liver, and spleen take up colloids to varying degrees, depending on particle size. The marrow most efficiently traps particles that are less than 1 μ in diameter. The ideal particle size range for spleen uptake is more than 1 μ in diameter; the liver most effectively takes up intermediate-sized particles. Tc-99m-sulfur colloid, a commonly used agent for imaging the RES, has particle diameters from 0.1 to 2.0 μ. The blood clearance half-time is about 3 minutes, so imaging can take place 15 to 20 minutes after injec-

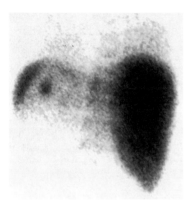

Figure 5–22. Accessory spleen. This posterior view of a Tc-99m-sulfur colloid image shows a small focus of increased uptake in the left upper quadrant adjacent to the normal spleen.

tion. About 90% of the injected tracer is taken up by the liver, 5% by the spleen, and 5% by the marrow.

Noncolloidal spleen imaging agents include labeled damaged red blood cells (RBCs) and labeled platelets. Heat-damaged RBCs are taken up by the spleen but not by the liver or the marrow. Tc-99m-damaged RBCs are thus useful for imaging splenic tissue that may be obscured by the liver in Tc-99m-SC imaging. This tracer can be used to locate and evaluate accessory spleens (Fig. 5–22), an aberrant spleen, or autotransplanted splenic tissue in patients who have undergone splenectomy following trauma. In-111-labeled platelets can be used to evaluate hypersplenism as a possible cause of thrombocytopenia.

Diffusely Increased Uptake

Increased uptake of colloidal tracers in the spleen relative to the liver occurs in patients with diffuse liver disease such as **cirrhosis** (Fig. 5–9). Diffuse liver disease usually affects both Kupffer cells and hepatocytes, so the increased colloid uptake by the spleen in diffuse liver disease is an indirect indicator of hepatocyte dysfunction. Increased splenic uptake of colloidal tracers in the face of normal liver function has been reported in patients with distant infections and tumors. However, the intensity of the spleen in the posterior view can be considerably greater than that of the liver in normals, so this sign should be interpreted with caution.

Figure 5–23. Lacerated spleen. Left lateral (upper left), left anterior oblique (upper right), left posterior oblique (lower left), and posterior (lower right) views. A photon-deficient band traverses the waist of the spleen in a person who experienced abdominal trauma. These findings are suggestive of a hematoma associated with a splenic laceration.

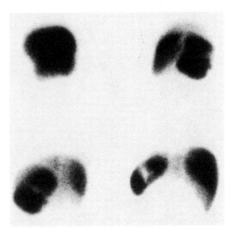

Focal Defects

Unlike other modalities, colloid spleen scintigraphy imaging permits the differentiation of functioning from nonfunctioning splenic tissue. Tc-99m-sulfur colloid imaging has proved to be very accurate in the diagnosis of **splenic lacerations** (Fig. 5–23). The findings typically consist of one or more defects that are often bandlike. The sensitivity and specificity of the test are both greater than 95%, and the positive predictive value is about 95%. The procedure is also useful in demonstrating other causes of focal splenic abnormalities such as abscesses, tumors, and infarcts.

Pancreas

Acute pancreatitis is usually diagnosed from the physical examination and laboratory data. In-111-leukocyte imaging is useful, however, in selecting patients who are unlikely to respond to conservative therapy. In one study all patients with negative scintigraphy at presentation improved with conservative therapy and were discharged. Forty-two percent of the patients with positive studies developed serious complications or died.

Pancreas transplantation in patients with severe complications of diabetes mellitus is becoming increasingly common. A major therapeutic problem in this setting is the early detection of rejection. Scintigraphic approaches to this problem have used Tc-99m-sulfur colloid, In-111-labeled platelets, and Tc-99m-DTPA.

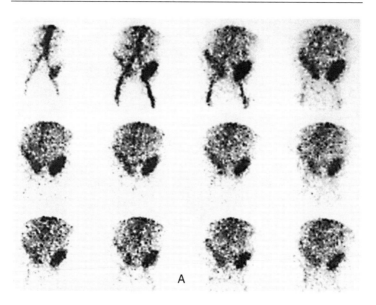

A

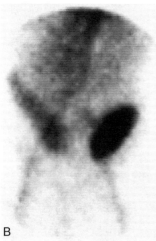

B

Figure 5–24. Normally functioning pancreas transplant. Two-second serial anterior perfusion images **(A)** and an immediate static anterior image **(B)** clearly delineate a pancreas of expected size and shape in the right side of the pelvis. A left pelvic renal transplant is also apparent.

The mechanism of Tc-99m-sulfur colloid uptake in malfunctioning pancreatic transplants is unknown but has been shown to correlate with diffuse small-vessel thrombosis. In-111-labeled platelets also become deposited in small thrombosed vessels.

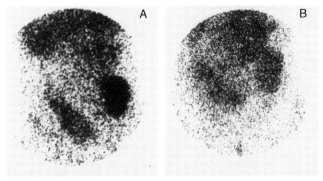

Figure 5–25. Pancreatitis in a transplant. Selected anterior images from rapid sequence perfusion studies 1 day following transplant **(A)** and several weeks later **(B)** show apparent enlargement and worsening of the definition of the transplanted pancreas in the right side of the pelvis. These findings suggest rejection or pancreatitis.

Imaging with either agent is a sensitive test for abnormal transplant function. However, conditions other than rejection, such as pancreatitis, atrophy, and infarction, also lead to positive results.

Imaging with Tc-99m-DTPA is convenient because this renal tracer is frequently used to study concomitant renal transplants (Fig. 5–24). Complications of the transplant are indicated by no perfusion or by a progressive increase in the apparent size of the transplant with an associated diminution in the distinctness of the transplant borders (Fig. 5–25). As in the other methods, this approach is reasonably sensitive but is not specific for rejection.

Suggested Readings

Brown PH, Juni JE, Lieberman DA, Krishnamurthy GT: Hepatocyte versus biliary disease: a distinction by deconvolutional analysis of technetium-99m IDA time–activity curves. *J Nucl Med* 1988;29: 623–630.

Budihna N, Milcinski M, Heberle J: Long-term follow-up after heterotopic splenic autotransplantation for traumatic splenic rupture. *J Nucl Med* 1991;32:204–207.

Bushnell DL, Perlman SB, Wilson MA, Polcyn RE: The rim sign: association with acute cholecystitis. *J Nucl Med* 1986;27:353–356.

Desai AG, Thakur ML: Radiopharmaceuticals for spleen and bone marrow studies. *Semin Nucl Med* 1985;13:229.

Doo E, Krishnamurthy GT, Eklem MJ, Gilbert S, Brown PH: Quantification of hepatobiliary function as an integral part of imaging with technetium-99m-mebrofenin in health and disease. *J Nucl Med* 1991;32:48–57.

Fig LM, Wahl RL, Stewart RE, Shapiro B: Morphine-augmented hepatobiliary scintigraphy in the severely ill: caution is in order. *Radiology* 1990;175:467–473.

Fink-Bennett D: Augmented cholescintigraphy: its role in detecting acute and chronic disorders of the hepatobiliary tree. *Semin Nucl Med* 1991;21:128–139.

Fink-Bennett D, Balon H, Robbins T, Tsai D: Morphine-augmented cholescintigraphy: its efficacy in detecting acute cholecystitis. *J Nucl Med* 1991;32:1231–1233.

Gambhir SS, Hawkins RA, Huang S-C, Hall TR, Busuttil RW, Phelps ME: Tracer kinetic modeling approaches for the quantification of hepatic function with technetium-99m DISIDA and scintigraphy. *J Nucl Med* 1989;30:1507–1518.

Gerhold JP, Klingensmith III WC, Kuni CC, et al: Diagnosis of biliary atresia with radionuclide hepatobiliary imaging. *Radiology* 1983;146:499–504.

Kim EE, Pjura G, Lowry P, Nguyen M, Pollack M: Morphine-augmented cholescintigraphy in the diagnosis of acute cholecystitis. *AJR* 1986;147:1177–1179.

Klingensmith WC III, Spitzer VM, Fritzberg AR, Kuni CC: The normal fasting and postprandial diisopropyl-IDA Tc99m hepatobiliary study. *Radiology* 1981;141:771–776.

Klingensmith WC III, Spitzer VM, Fritzberg AR, Kuni CC: Normal appearance and reproducibility of liver-spleen studies with Tc-99m sulfur colloid and Tc-99m microalbumin colloid. *J Nucl Med* 1983;24:8–13.

Kloiber R, AuCoin R, Hershfield NB, et al: Biliary obstruction after cholecystectomy: diagnosis with quantitative cholescintigraphy. *Radiology* 1988;169:643–647.

Kudo M, Ikekubo K, Yamamoto K, et al: Distinction between hemangioma of the liver and hepatocellular carcinoma: value of labeled RBC-SPECT scanning. *AJR* 1989;152:977–983.

Kuni C, Klingensmith WC, Fritzberg AR: Evaluation of intrahepatic cholestasis with radionuclide hepatobiliary imaging. *Gastrointest Radiol* 1984;9:163–166.

Kuni CC, Klingensmith WC: *Atlas of Radionuclide Hepatobiliary Imaging.* Boston: GK Hall, 1983;147–165.

Lubbers PR, Ros PR, Goodman ZD, Ishak KG: Accumulation of technetium-99m sulfur colloid by hepatocellular adenoma: scintigraphic-pathologic correlation. *AJR* 1987;148:1105–1108.

Nagle CE, Freitas J, Dworkin HJ: Cholescintigraphy in Cholecystic Cancer. *Clinical Nuclear Medicine* 1983;8:220–222.

Nelson RC, Chezmar JL: Diagnostic approach to hepatic hemangiomas. *Radiology* 1990;176:11–13.

Smith R, Rosen JM, Gallo LN, Alderson PO: Pericholecystic hepatic activity in cholescintigraphy. *Radiology* 1985;156:797–800.

Spencer RP, Gupta SM: Radionuclide studies of the spleen in trauma and iatrogenic disorders. *Semin Nucl Med* 1985;15:305.

Swayne LC: Acute acalculous cholecystitis: sensitivity in detection using technetium-99m iminodiacetic acid cholescintigraphy. *Radiology* 1986;160:33–38.

Weissmann HS, Badia J, Sugarman LA, Kluger L, Rosenblatt R, Freeman LM: Spectrum of 99m-Tc-IDA cholescintigraphic patterns in acute cholecystitis. *Radiology* 1981;138:167–175.

Yap L, Wycherley AG, Morphett AD, Toouli J: Acalculous biliary pain: cholecystectomy alleviates symptoms in patients with abnormal cholescintigraphy. *Gastroenterology* 1991;101:786–793.

Chapter 6

Genitourinary System

Radiopharmaceuticals

Choosing the best radiopharmaceutical for evaluation of the genitourinary system demands familiarity with products that are now available. Once there is an understanding of what the referring clinician needs to know, it is possible to gain functional or morphologic information. Basic knowledge of renal physiology is the starting point for selecting the best scintigraphic method.

The total perfusion of the kidney is represented by the renal plasma flow. Only 20% of this plasma flow is filtered through the semipermeable membrane of the glomerulus. The filtrate that is protein-free is then nearly completely reabsorbed in the tubules. The glomerular filtration rate (GFR) quantitates the amount of filtrate formed per minute. Autoregulation by the kidney maintains filtration during a range of arterial pressures. The classic agent for determining GFR is inulin, which once filtered is not reabsorbed or secreted. The concentration of inulin in glomerular filtrate reflects the concentration of inulin within plasma. Plasma clearance of inulin is therefore a function of urine volume and concentration of inulin relative to plasma concentration. Normal GFR in adults is approximately 125 mL/min. Radiopharmaceuticals that have been successfully used to assess GFR have included I-125 iothalamate and, since 1970, Tc-99m-DTPA (diethylenetriamine penta-acetic acid). Results for GFR calculated by DTPA are generally acceptable, although 5 to 10% of injected DTPA is protein-bound. Assessment of GFR by Tc-99m-DTPA has advantages over creatinine clearance because in disease states tubular secretion of creatinine may significantly increase. Scintigraphic techniques also allow some degree of assessment of relative GFR for each kidney, which is not possible by creatinine clearance.

An agent that is completely cleared from the blood by the kidney would be ideal for measuring effective renal plasma flow. Para-amino hippuric acid (PAH) has been the classic agent to measure effective renal plasma flow (ERPF), yielding a normal value of 585 mL/min in adults. Measurement of ERPF by scintigraphic techniques has been possible since formulation of iodine-131-OIH. The clearance of OIH is approximately 15% lower than that of PAH. Measurements of GFR and ERPF are thus possible by use of Tc-99m-DTPA and I-131-OIH, respectively.

Methods to assess GFR and ERPF have used compartmental and imaging models. Imaging methods have been applied to quantitate relative renal function by comparing tracer uptake in each kidney during an early period after injection. Split function quantitation should take place generally during the 1- to 3-minute interval after injection and before activity has appeared in the collecting system. Image-based methods to assess DTPA filtration are based on assumptions relating the ratio of renal counts to the injected dose. Correction factors must account for attenuation by soft tissue between the camera and the cardiac blood pool and kidneys. In general, imaging methods to quantitate renal function are prone to large errors. The most accurate method for determining disappearance of a radiopharmaceutical from the blood would construct a multiexponential plasma disappearance curve by obtaining multiple blood samples after injection. This method is too demanding for routine clinical work and has now given way at most institutions to the method of Tauxe, which allows measurement of ERPF from a single plasma sample at 44 minutes after injection of OIH. There is good correlation in adults between the single 44-minute sample technique and the multiple sample technique. However, the method is not as reliable in children or in patients with prominent extravascular fluid collections such as ascites, edema, or peritoneal dialysis fluid. GFR is best quantitated by obtaining blood samples 2 to 4 hours after injection. To obtain a volume of distribution the plasma disappearance curve is then extrapolated to the time of injection. Once volume of distribution is known, plasma clearance is obtained by multiplying the volume of distribution times the slope of the plasma disappearance curve.

The number of radiopharmaceutical products available for routine imaging of the kidneys remains bewildering to even relatively experienced referring clinicians and is the subject of frequent radiologic consultation. Tc-99m-pertechnetate is an overall poor choice for routine imaging because 85% of filtered radiopharmaceutical is reabsorbed by the tubules. Pertechne-

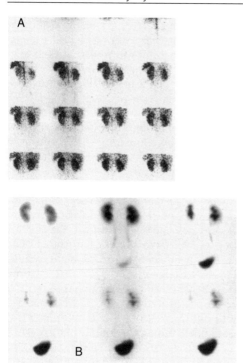

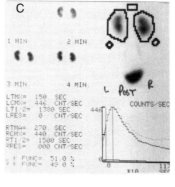

Figure 6–1. Normal Tc-99m-DTPA renogram. **(A)** The perfusion phase framed at 2 seconds per image shows prompt and symmetric perfusion of the kidneys. **(B)** The dynamic functional phase is framed at 3 minutes per image and shows symmetric cortical activity in the first image and prompt appearance of the collecting system by the second image. The collecting system is well visualized and is unremarkable. **(C)** The renogram curve for Tc-99m-DTPA should normally peak between 3 and 5 minutes as it does here. An approximate quantitation of relative renal function can be obtained from an image obtained prior to 3 minutes before the collecting system is visualized. Other quantitative numbers may be generated but should never be used in isolation without viewing the dynamic functional images.

tate's use in the genitourinary system is primarily for testicular scanning and for detection of vesicoureteral reflux.

Tc-99m-DTPA has been a mainstay for assessment of glomerular filtration by imaging methods. It is well suited to imaging because only 5 to 10% is protein bound and approximately 5% remains in the kidneys 4 hours following injection. More than 90% is excreted by filtration and is not reabsorbed. Use of Tc-99m as the isotope provides useful delineation of parenchymal and collecting system anatomy (Fig. 6–1).

In the past, renal excretory function was best studied with OIH. The extraction efficiency of OIH is nearly 90% and is better than that of any Tc-99m-labeled agents. Eighty percent of excretion is by tubular transport, and 20% is by glomerular filtration. Blood clearance is therefore faster than that for any filtration agent, and diagnostic studies may be obtained in kidneys where function has been impaired down to 3% of normal levels. The significant trade-offs for these benefits are the poor imaging characteristics of I-131. The attempt to solve this problem with I-123-OIH was compromised by the short shelf life and high cost of I-123.

These challenges were surmounted when Tc-99m-MAG$_3$ became routinely available for imaging. The rates at which OIH and MAG$_3$ appear in the urine are nearly identical. Although Tc-99m-MAG$_3$ is more heavily protein bound than OIH, relatively more remains in the intravascular space and is available for clearance by the kidney. The overall biological properties of MAG$_3$ and OIH are similar, and renogram curves can be interpreted in the same general manner. When correction factors are utilized, Tc-99m-MAG$_3$ provides ERPF assessments that are in agreement with data obtained with OIH. Tc-99m-MAG$_3$, because of its combination of OIH-like biological properties and favorable imaging characteristics, has therefore become the most promising radiopharmaceutical product for routine renal imaging (Fig. 6–2).

Tc-99m-DMSA is a useful cortical imaging tracer that provides a detailed examination of functioning tubular mass. Approximately 40 to 60% remains bound to the proximal tubules at 3 to 6 hours following injection. DMSA is heavily protein bound and is thus minimally filtered through the glomerulus. However, target-to-background ratios remain high, providing excellent morphologic cortical detail. Imaging is possible during states of renal failure, when scans may be delayed up

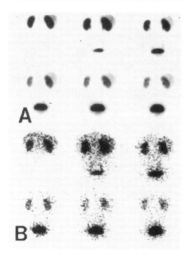

Figure 6–2. Comparison of imaging with Tc-99m-MAG₃ and I-131 hippuran. This patient was simultaneously injected with **(A)** Tc-99m-MAG₃ and **(B)** I-131 hippuran. The favorable imaging properties of Tc-99m-MAG₃ are readily apparent when imaging is performed using separate energy windows. The high photon flux obtained with Tc-99m-MAG₃ produces better delineation of the renal cortex and collecting system. Faint hepatic activity may occasionally be seen as in this patient. No abnormality is visualized on this study.

to 24 hours after injection. Sulfhydril binding to the tubules defines DMSA as a predominantly anatomic agent (Fig. 6–3).

Tc-99m-glucoheptonate is a compromise between the physiologic properties of DTPA and DMSA. Approximately 30 to 45% of this carbohydrate is excreted by glomerular filtration within

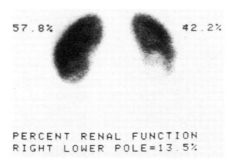

57.8%   42.2%

PERCENT RENAL FUNCTION
RIGHT LOWER POLE=13.5%

Figure 6–3. Tc-99m-DMSA renal imaging. Note the high target-to-background ratio of activity with absence of tracer within the collecting system. There is mild loss of cortex in the left lower pole and more significant loss of renal cortex in the right lower pole. In this patient with bilateral vesicoureteral reflux DMSA imaging is ideally suited to quantitation of relative renal activity because of the relative lack of background and collecting system activity.

the first hour. Five to 15% of the remaining product remains bound to the renal tubules. Cortical images can thus be obtained at 1 to 4 hours following injection in a manner similar to that of DMSA. There is significant visualization of the biliary system, and this can interfere with assessment of functioning tubular mass. Because of tubular binding, radiation doses to the kidney for glucoheptonate and DMSA are higher than those for DTPA.

Renal imaging is done to assess renal perfusion, cortical abnormalities, and excretory function. The patient is placed in the supine position to allow the kidneys to be equidistant from the collimator. A bolus of radiopharmaceutical is injected and subsequent images are obtained at 1- to 5-second intervals. Once the bolus reaches the abdominal aorta, symmetrical visualization of peak renal activity should take place within approximately 6 seconds of peak aortic activity, assuming an adequate bolus was injected. Time–activity curves are then obtained over the kidneys with the region of interest placed over the whole kidney or the cortex. Peak cortical activity is at 3 to 5 minutes following Tc-99m-DTPA injection and at 2 to 3 minutes following injection of I-131 hippuran or Tc-99m-MAG$_3$. The renogram curve is generally divided into a rising phase that describes concentration or tracer extraction (uptake) and a declining phase that describes tracer excretion. The curve begins to decline when excretion exceeds tracer extraction. Dehydration will cause some delay of peak of the renogram curve and some flattening of the excretory phase. Ideally, all patients should be well hydrated. Protocols to ensure this are of special importance for patients undergoing evaluation for obstruction.

Interpretation

Various methods have been described to aid in interpretation of the renogram. Deconvolution analysis has been applied in some centers to give a more accurate renal transit time of the injected radiopharmaceutical. Although it corrects for dispersion of the bolus and recirculation, it has not seen widespread application for routine imaging. Numerical data obtained by interpretation of the renogram are aided considerably by the higher count rates achieved with a Tc-99m agent. Values generated by quantitative analysis should be interpreted in conjunction with visual interpretation of the renogram.

Use of Tc-99m-labeled agents allows the visual assessment of

vesicoureteral reflux. By the indirect method the radiopharmaceutical is injected intravenously and 1 to 2 hours are allowed for bladder filling and clearance of activity from the kidneys. The patient must not void during this period, and subsequent sequential imaging is performed to assess the presence of reflux during voiding. By this method catheterization is avoided and functional information can be obtained. In approximately 20% of cases there is reflux during filling of the bladder, and this finding would be missed by the indirect method. The direct method is therefore most commonly applied. A Foley catheter is placed in the bladder and 0.5 to 1.0 mCi of Tc-99m-pertechnetate, DTPA, or sulfur colloid are instilled. The catheter is connected to a bottle of normal saline that is suspended no more than 100 cm above the table, and the patient is imaged in the supine position with a gamma camera beneath the table. Care is taken to avoid contamination of the table and the collimator. Although imaging is continuous, framing rates may vary from 5 to 30 seconds per image. Image intensity should be optimized to detect small amounts of ureteral reflux. Continuous acquisition continues when the patient voids around the catheter or after the catheter is removed. The volume at which reflux begins should be noted. Optional techniques include the measurement of intravesicle pressures using a double-lumen catheter and the quantitation of residual bladder volume. Radiation dose to the bladder is approximately 30 mrad, which is an order of magnitude less than that obtained during a radiographic VCUG. The radiographic VCUG remains the test of choice for initial diagnostic evaluation to grade the degree of reflux and to describe collecting system morphology. The radionuclide technique is more sensitive and, because of a lower radiation dose, is better suited to sequential follow-up (Fig. 6–4).

Diuretic augmented renography is well suited to differentiation of the **obstructed and nonobstructed dilated collecting system.** Findings depend on the nature, duration, and severity of obstruction. In high-grade acute obstructions that have been present for several days there is a noticeable delay in renal perfusion. Severity and duration of obstruction affect the concentration and excretion phases of the renogram. Early images of the kidney may show a photon-deficient defect in the region of the collecting system, with gradual accumulation of activity. Some conclusions can be drawn about the shape and size of the col-

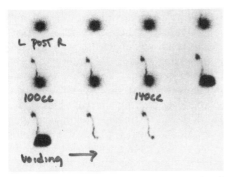

Figure 6–4. Positive left vesicoureteral reflux. This study is divided into 10-second frames and is performed with Tc-99m-sulfur colloid in normal saline. Left-sided reflux occurs into the intrarenal collecting system with installation of 100 mL of normal saline. As was the case here this study is continued until the drip of normal saline slows considerably or there is voiding. Imaging during voiding is important because reflux may occur during this phase.

lecting system and the site of obstruction at this early point, although caution must be exercised in assigning a specific degree of collecting system dilation with radionuclide studies. Patients who have sufficient activity within the collecting system can be evaluated following intravenous injection of 0.3 to 1.0 mg/kg dose of furosemide. The patient should empty the bladder prior to intravenous injection of diuretic. A Foley catheter should be in place in the pediatric patient. Time–activity curves generated following diuretic administration can then give some indication about the degree of obstruction. The diuretic effect takes place almost immediately following injection, although a peak effect is not reached for approximately 10 minutes. In nonobstructed systems there is a prompt drop in activity in the region of interest over the renal pelvis or whole kidney. When a line is extrapolated using the most rapid response, a half-time of clearance can be obtained. Nonobstructed kidneys generally have a half-time of less than 10 minutes, whereas with significant obstruction the half-times are greater than 20 minutes. Markedly atonic dilated systems or impaired states of renal function may obscure the result and lead to further interventional testing by nonscintigraphic techniques. The most frequent application of diuretic renography is in the pediatric population. Causes of the **uretero-**

pelvic junction (UPJ) obstruction in the pediatric population include ureteral recanalization failure, mucosal folds or hypertrophy, fibrosis or atresia, extrarenal pelves with angulations or kinks, and fibrous bands or crossing vessels. Patients who have undergone UPJ repairs can be evaluated in the early postoperative state to assess the degree of surgical success before ultrasound shows any change in the collecting system (Fig. 6–5). Whitaker invasive pressure/perfusion testing is no longer popular in this population and significant emphasis is now placed on the scintigraphic results. When there is a question of distal or midureteral obstruction, regions of interest can be drawn over the ureter during diuretic renography. Patients should be well hydrated prior to examination to prevent low urine flow rates in a nonobstructive system. Diuretic renography is not helpful when there is no significant collecting system activity prior to furosemide administration. Delayed images are better suited to this population.

Scintigraphic studies are occasionally applied to detect **renal artery stenosis.** Standard scintigraphic techniques involving flow and function measurements are insufficient to detect renovascular disease, but an angiotensin-converting enzyme (ACE) inhibitor can allow differentiation between the normal and the affected kidney. By preventing the production of angiotensin II, an ACE inhibitor such as captopril or enalapril prevents vasoconstriction of the efferent arteriole. During states of significant renal artery stenosis glomerular perfusion pressure is maintained by efferent arteriolar constriction. Glomerular filtration is thus maintained in the setting of decreased renal perfusion. Although a variety of radiopharmaceuticals—including DMSA, MAG_3, and OIH—are being evaluated for use with captopril renography, DTPA remains a good indicator of decreased glomerular filtration following captopril administration. A dose of 25 to 50 mg of captopril is given 1 hour prior to administration of Tc-99m-DTPA. Blood pressure should be monitored for systemic hypotension. A physician should be available to hydrate the patient if necessary. A qualitative change from a baseline DTPA renogram is then used for evaluation. The change in the renogram does not necessarily correspond to the degree of renal artery stenosis. If significant renal artery stenosis is present, one typically sees decreased uptake of DTPA, delay in time to maximal activity, and delay in cortical washout (Fig. 6–6). For evalu-

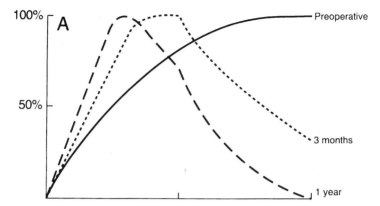

Figure 6–5. Pre- and postoperative scintigraphy for ureteral pelvic junction obstruction. Significant improvement is seen in the renogram pattern at 3 months and 1 year following surgery. Ultrasound examinations revealed persistent hydronephrosis.

ation of unilateral renal artery stenosis, sensitivity greater than 90% can be expected with captopril renography. In bilateral renal artery stenosis the test is limited but can document the more severely involved kidney. The future application of the test will be to identify patients who will optimally respond to treatment by angioplasty or surgery.

Tc-99m-DMSA is well suited to the evaluation of differential renal function in a patient who is about to undergo renal resection or revascularization. Although the activity in the early phase of a DTPA renogram can be used as an indicator of relative function, the most accurate results are obtained by relative uptake of DMSA. DMSA distribution correlates strongly with differential glomerular filtration and differential renal blood flow. The overall representation is that of viable nephron mass. The relative activity should be averaged from anterior and posterior acquisitions.

Another cost-efficient use of Tc-99m-DMSA is the evaluation of **pseudotumors** of the kidney. Developmental variants such as columns of Bertin, dromedary humps, and fetal lobulations can be shown to be composed of normal renal parenchyma. The evaluation of all other intrarenal masses is usually by other diagnostic techniques. In children **Wilms' tumor** may occasionally be

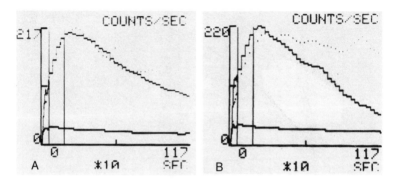

Figure 6–6. Renal artery stenosis. **(A)** Symmetric renogram patterns are seen prior to captopril administration. **(B)** One hour following the oral administration of 25 mg of captopril there is a unilateral abnormality in the renogram curve (dotted line) that correlates with proven renal artery stenosis.

evaluated using serial DMSA scans, although detection is limited to lesions that are greater than 1 cm in diameter. Another good pediatric application of DMSA is the evaluation of **horseshoe kidneys** or **crossed fused ectopia** (Fig. 6–7).

Infections that are intrarenal, perinephric, and paranephric can occasionally be diagnosed by radionuclide tests. Diffuse infections characteristically result in decreased perfusion and abnormalities of the renogram curve. **Acute pyelonephritis**, when seen with DMSA, will sometimes show photon-deficient defects that appear to radiate from the pelvicalyceal system into various portions of the cortex. The affected kidney may be enlarged or normal in size. The best application of cortical imaging tracers is for focal infections of the kidney. Examination by intravenous urography or ultrasonography is generally not as sensitive as cortical imaging in the pediatric population. The advantage of DMSA scanning in children is further enhanced by favorable dosimetry, avoidance of contrast injection or bowel preparation, and lack of degradation by overlying bowel gas. An additional benefit is the assessment of relative renal function. There is a complimentary role for gallium-67 citrate if the clinician is willing to wait at least 24 hours to evaluate the kidney. Indium-111 leukocytes localize in renal infections, increasing the

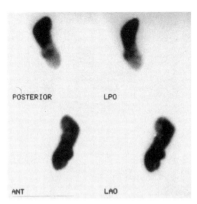

POSTERIOR   LPO

ANT   LAO

Figure 6–7. Crossed fused renal ectopia. Tc-99m-DMSA is useful for cortical delineation of developmental variants or aberrant renal tissue. Quantitation of the upper and lower components of this fused renal mass would be possible from the anterior and posterior images.

specificity of photon-deficient defect seen with cortical imaging tracers. Tc-99m-DMSA should be considered in patients with fever of unknown origin or in patients when upper and lower urinary tract infections cannot be easily differentiated.

Complications of **renal transplantation** are often identified using scintigraphic techniques during the immediate and extended period following transplantation. Combined immunosuppressive therapy now includes prednisone, cyclosporine, azathioprine, and antilymphocyte globulin, and OKT3 for cadaveric transplant recipients. The nephrotoxic effects of cyclosporine that were commonly seen in the early 1980s are not as frequent now. Methods of evaluation include use of Tc-99m-DTPA, Tc-99m-MAG$_3$, or simultaneous administration of I-131 OIH and Tc-99m-DTPA. The assessment of renal cortical perfusion requires administration of a relatively compact bolus of either Tc-99m-DTPA or -MAG$_3$. Perfusion of the transplant is considered normal when time between peak iliac artery activity and peak transplant activity is 6 to 8 seconds. Various hyperemic anatomic structures such as proliferative endometrium and normal bowel and mesentery may appear as normal variants on the flow phase (Fig. 6–8). Abnormalities seen during perfusion evaluation can be evaluated with Tc-99m-DMSA for improved anatomic definition (Fig. 6–9). Captopril testing is possible in the renal transplant recipient when there is a question of renal artery stenosis involving the allograft. Possible inhibitory effects between cyclosporine and captopril may complicate evaluation. Quantitative methods to evaluate glomerular filtration rate and

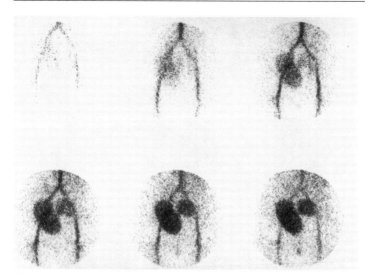

Figure 6–8. A normal variant on flow phase. Hyperemic endometrium may occasionally appear as a normal structure during the perfusion phase of a Tc-99m-DTPA or Tc-99m-MAG$_3$ renogram.

ERPF as described previously can be applied to the renal transplant recipient.

Postoperative fluid collections are best evaluated using DTPA or MAG$_3$. **Urinomas** are of the greatest consequence and show

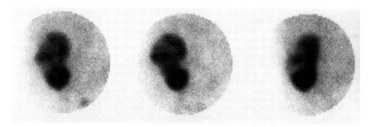

Figure 6–9. Renal cortical infarcts. Wedge-shaped perfusion abnormalities are present in this right-sided pelvic renal transplant following injection of Tc-99m-DMSA. Projections include the anterior, right anterior oblique, and left lateral views showing the infarcts to be primarily in the upper and middle portions of the kidney and primarily anterior. These abnormalities corresponded to an angiographically proven arterial occlusion.

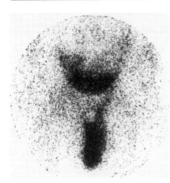

Figure 6–10. Scrotal urinoma. Gradual accumulation of Tc-99m-DTPA was seen in this patient with scrotal swelling. The ultrasound study revealed indistinct anatomic planes but no discrete fluid collections.

gradual accumulation of tracer on delayed images (Fig. 6–10). A bladder catheter is helpful to prevent obscuration of **urine leak** or urinoma by bladder activity. **Intraperitoneal leaks** can be demonstrated by tracer accumulation with an anatomic site such as the paracolic gutters or the subphrenic space (Fig. 6–11). **Lymphoceles** will appear as photon-deficient defects within weeks or months following transplantations (Fig. 6–12). Delayed tracer accumulation should not occur within these fluid collections. The evalua-

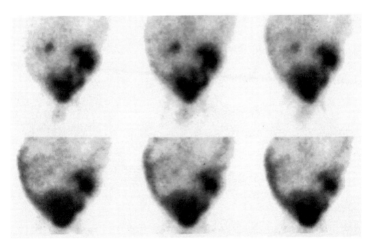

Figure 6–11. Intraperitoneal urine leak. Renograms are highly sensitive for detection of postoperative complications such as intraperitoneal urine leaks. In this patient progressive appearance of the right paracolic gutter is diagnostic of urine leak.

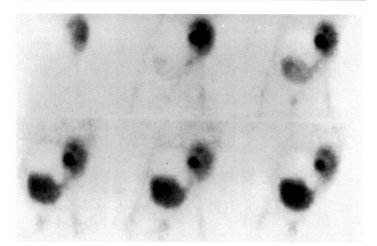

Figure 6–12. Lymphocele. A photon-deficient abnormality is seen superior to the bladder and shows no accumulation of Tc-99m-DTPA. Accumulation of Tc-99m-DTPA would be expected if this had been a urinoma.

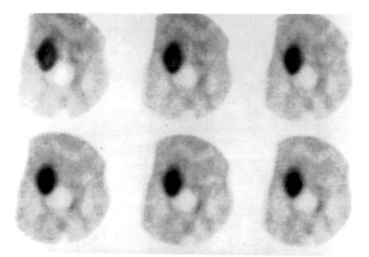

Figure 6–13. Partially obstructing lymphocele. This lymphocele is in a common location between the transplant kidney and the bladder and was noted to stretch and deviate the ureter. Partial obstruction is suggested by retention of tracer within the pelvis of the kidney. There is minimal accumulation of tracer within the bladder, which has been displaced toward the patient's left side.

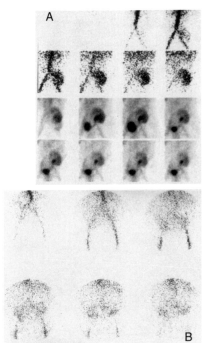

Figure 6–14. Normal transplant flow and functional study. **(A)** In a normal transplant renogram the peak cortical activity is seen within 6 to 8 seconds of the adjoining peak iliac arterial activity peak. Appearance of the tracer within the collecting system is seen during the second 3-minute frame of the functional phase of the renogram. Note that bladder emptying has occurred during the functional phase of the study. **(B)** In this patient with acute rejection there is markedly diminished flow to the new left-sided renal transplant. The previous right-sided transplant is also indistinct and poorly perfused.

tion of **ureteral obstruction** can be achieved with furosemide administration using either quantitative or qualitative interpretation. Visual assessment of the degree of obstruction is usually sufficient (Fig. 6–13). In the immediate posttransplantation period there may be relatively prominent visualization of the ureter because of edema at the ureterovesicle anastomosis.

Although considerable effort has been expended to differentiate **rejection** from other causes of allograft dysfunction, there is no reliable method that does not require significant clinical input (Fig. 6–14). Specialized techniques involving indium-111-labeled platelets and iodine-125-labeled fibrinogen remain problematic at best. Persistent gallium-67 citrate uptake in the allograft has also been found to be nonspecific. **Cyclosporine** toxicity and acute rejection cannot be differentiated reliably. Cyclosporine effects usually occur later, following transplantation, such as in the 2- to 3-month period rather than in the first 30 days. Cyclosporine toxicity is associated

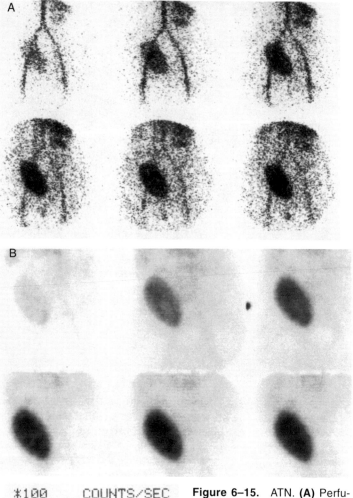

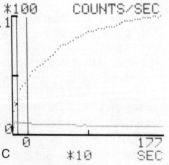

Figure 6–15. ATN. **(A)** Perfusion to the renal transplant is typically unremarkable during uncomplicated ATN. **(B)** A progressive cortical accumulation pattern with no visible excretion on this Tc-99m-MAG$_3$ study is the most commonly encountered pattern following ATN. **(C)** A rising renogram pattern is compatible with but not specific for ATN.

with cyclosporine trough levels that are greater than 200 mg/mL.

Sequential combined isotope studies are helpful in the evaluation of the transplant recipient. Studies obtained during periods of normal function are helpful in documenting the onset and resolution of abnormalities in perfusion, tubular function, and glomerular filtration. **Acute tubular necrosis (ATN)** is much more common in cadaveric transplants and should be suspected when relatively normal perfusion and markedly abnormal uptake and excretion exist in the first week following transplantation. Because there is usually severely compromised glomerular filtration during episodes of ATN, the allograft may barely be seen above background levels on a DTPA study (Fig. 6–15). Studies using I-131 hippuran or Tc-99m-MAG$_3$ may show slow gradual accumulation of cortical activity with little or no visible excretion (Fig. 6–16). Acute tubulointerstitial or acute vascular rejection episodes usually do not occur before 4 or 5 days following transplantation. The classic appearance of an acute rejection episode shows moderately or markedly impaired perfusion with associated poor uptake and delayed excretion. Chronic rejection is the end result of multiple episodes of failed immunosuppression and therefore follows multiple episodes of acute rejection.

Tc-99m-MAG$_3$ allows evaluation of perfusion and tubular function while giving excellent anatomic detail of the kidney and collecting system. MAG$_3$ will give better diagnostic quality than DTPA during states of impaired renal function (Fig. 6–17). The spatial resolution obtained with this technetium agent provides better anatomic detail than that obtained with OIH.

Scrotal imaging is requested when the clinician wants to differentiate **testicular torsion** from **epididymitis.** Perfusion of the scrotum is supplied by pudendal vessels that do not pass through the spermatic cord. When torsion occurs it is generally due to a congenital abnormality ("bell-clapper" deformity) where the testicle is free to rotate within the tunica vaginalis. Perfusion of the scrotum is not compromised with testicular torsion. Pudendal vessels do not supply collaterals to the arteries of the spermatic cord. Salvage of the affected testicle is high when the diagnosis of torsion is made within 5 to 6 hours. Although epididymitis may be clinically indistinguishable from torsion, a flow study will show increased perfusion through the spermatic cord. Increased tracer activity is usually seen in the region of the epididymitis and a reactive hydrocele may be present (Fig. 6–19). This sensitivity of testicular

Figure 6–16. Tc-99m-DTPA versus I-131 hippuran in ATN. This patient simultaneously received Tc-99m-DTPA (above) and I-131 hippuran (below). In severe ATN the Tc-99m-DTPA study may show little filtration and therefore little distinction of the renal transplant from the background activity. More diagnostic information is obtained from the progressive cortical accumulation pattern seen with I-131 hippuran, because residual tubular transport allows differentiation of the transplant from the background.

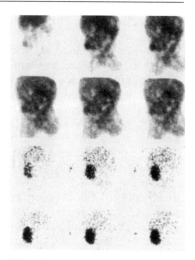

Figure 6–17. Comparison of Tc-99m-MAG$_3$ and I-131 hippuran. This patient simultaneously received Tc-99m-DTPA **(A)** and I-131 hippuran **(B).** The marked difference in resolution obtained with the Tc-99m study allows visualization of significantly more anatomic detail, such as this small bladder diverticulum.

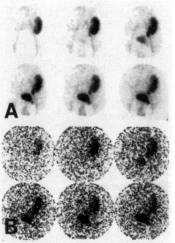

scintigraphy for the detection of torsion is high when properly performed. A bolus of 10 to 20 mCi of Tc-99m-pertechnetate is injected and a series of 3- to 5-second images are required. A lead–rubber shield is then placed behind the scrotum and a 500,000-count image is obtained following the angiographic phase. The study is limited in neonates when even pinhole collimation may not be of sufficient resolution. In acute torsion the

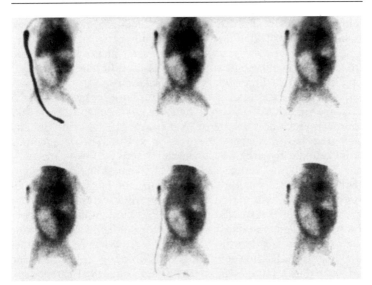

Figure 6–18. Arterial occlusion. The functional phase of this Tc-99m-DTPA renogram reveals the "punched hole" appearance of absent arterial perfusion of this right-sided renal transplant in a young patient.

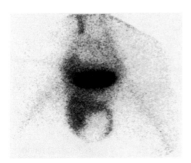

Figure 6–19. Testicular perfusion study. Following injection of Tc-99m pertechnetate there is increased perfusion to the right side of the scrotum suggestive of epididymitis. A photopenic defect seen on the left aspect of the scrotum is secondary to a reactive hydrocele.

testes will appear as a photon-deficient defect while dartos activity is normal. In late or **missed torsion** there is a prominent increase of perfusion of the dartos resulting in a bull's-eye appearance. This rim of hyperemic activity is not specific and may be seen with **hematoma** or **abscess**. If there is spontaneous detorsion there is usually return to a normal flow and static image pattern. Duplex Doppler sonography provides better anatomic detail and quantitative evaluation of flow and is now finding widespread application in the differential of acute scrotal pain.

Some applications of genitourinary scintigraphy are rare or require an investigational new-drug license. Iodine-131 iodomethyl 19-norcholesterol (NP-59) can be used in conjunction with dexamethasone suppression to differentiate **adenoma** from **adrenal hyperplasia.** Asymmetric activity favors the presence of adenoma. Iodine-123 or -131 metaiodobenzylguanidine (MIBG) is useful for **pheochromocytoma** or **metastatic neuroblastoma.** There is some evidence that MIBG scanning is slightly more sensitive and specific than skeletal scintigraphy in neuroblastoma patients. Somatostatin receptor studies with octreotide are becoming useful in this population even when MIBG studies are negative. Radionuclide hysterosalpingography has been advocated as a physiologic means of assessing tubal patency following installation of Tc-99m-labeled human albumin microspheres into the posterior vaginal fornix. Tc-99m-pertechnetate has been used to assess **penile vascular insufficiency** and response to vasodilator therapy.

Suggested Readings

Abramson SJ, et al: Diuretic renography in the assessment of urinary tract dilation in children. *Pediatr Radiol* 1983;13:319–323.

Beierwaltes WH: Clinical applications of[131]iodine-labeled metaiodobenzylguanidine. In: Hoffer PB, ed. *Yearbook of Nuclear Medicine.* Chicago: Year Book, 1987;17–34.

Bejjani B, Belman AB: Ureteropelvic junction obstruction in newborns and infants. *J Urol* 1982;128:770–773.

Captopril Symposium: *Am J Hypertens* 1992;4(12):661–740.

Chen DCP, Holder LE, Melloul M: Radionuclide scrotal imaging: further experience with 210 new patients. I. Anatomy, pathophysiology and methods. *J Nucl Med* 1983;24:735–742.

Chen DCP, Holder LE, Melloul M: Radionuclide scrotal imaging: further experience with 210 patients. II. Results and discussion. *J Nucl Med* 1983;24:841–853.

Conway JJ: Role of scintigraphy in urinary tract infection. *Semin Nucl Med* 1988;18:308–319.

Davidson RA, Wilcox CS: Newer tests for the diagnosis of renovascular disease. *JAMA* 1992;268(23):3353–3358.

Dondi M, Franchi R, Levorato M, et al: Evaluation of hypertensive patients by means of captopril enhanced renal scintigraphy with technetium-99m DTPA. *J Nucl Med* 1989;30:615–621.

Dondi M, Monetti N, Fanti S, et al: Use of technetium-99m-MAG$_3$ for renal scintigraphy after angiotensin-converting enzyme inhibition. *J Nucl Med* 1991;32:424–428.

Dubovsky EV, Russell CD: Radionuclide evaluation of renal transplants. *Semin Nucl Med* 1988;18:181–198.

duCret RP: Scintigraphic evaluation of the renal transplant recipient. In: Letourneau JG, Day DL, Ascher NL, eds. *Radiology Organtransplantation.* St Louis: Mosby Yearbook, 1991;83–98.

duCret RP, Boudreau RJ, Gonzalez R, Carpenter R, Tennison J, Kuni CC: Clinical efficacy of Tc-99m-MAG$_3$ kit formulation in routine renal scintigraphy. *J Urology* 1989;142:19–22.

Fine EJ: Interventions in renal scintigraphy. *Semin Nucl Med* 1991;21:116–127.

Fine EJ, Axelrod M, Gorkin J, et al: Measurement of effective renal plasma flow: a comparison of methods. *J Nucl Med* 1987;28:1393–1400.

Freeman LM, Blaufox MD, eds: Transplant evaluation. *Semin Nucl Med* 1988;18(3):181–198.

Goates JJ, Morton KA, Wooten WW, et al: Comparison of methods for calculating glomerular filtration rate: Tc-99m DTPA scintigraphic analysis, protein-free and whole plasma clearance of Tc-99m DTPA and I-125 iothalamate. *J Nucl Med* 1990;31:424–429.

Gordon I: Indications for 99m technetium dimercaptosuccinic acid scan in children. *J Urol* 1987;137:464–467.

Hilson AJW, Lewis CA: Radionuclide studies in impotence. *Semin Nucl Med* 1991;21:159–163.

Hosokawa S, et al: Congenital renal anomaly: evaluation with 99m-Tc-dimercaptosuccinic acid renal scintigraphy. *Am J Kidney Dis* 1983;2:655–659.

Kletter K, Nurnberger N: Diagnostic potential of diuresis renography: limitations by the severity of hydronephrosis and by impairment of renal function. *Nucl Med Commun* 1989;10:51–61.

Middleton WD, Siegel BA, Melson GL, Yates CK, Andriole GL: Acute scrotal disorders: prospective comparison of color Doppler US and testicular scintigraphy. *Radiology* 1990;177:177–181.

Nasrallah PF, Nara S, Crawford J: Clinical applications of nuclear cystography. *J Urol* 1982;128:550–553.

Russell CD, Dubovsky EV: Measurement of renal function with radionuclides. *J Nucl Med* 1989;30:2053–2057.

Russell CD, Thorstad BL, Stutzman ME, Yester MV, Fowler D,

Dubovsky EV: The kidney: imaging with Tc-99m mercaptoacetyl-triglycine, a technetium-labeled analog of iodohippurate. *Radiology* 1989;172:427–430.

Sfakianakis GN, Sfakianakis ED: Nuclear medicine in pediatric urology and nephrology. *J Nucl Med* 1988;29:1287–1300.

Sty JR, Starshak RJ, Hubbard AM: Radionuclide evaluation in childhood injuries. *Semin Nucl Med* 1983;13:258–281.

Tauxe WN, Dubovsky EV, Kidd T, et al: New formulas for the calculation of effective renal plasma flow. *Eur J Nucl Med* 1982;7:51–54.

Taylor A, Ziffer JA, Steves A, et al: Clinical comparison of I-131 OIH and the kit formulation of Tc-99m mercaptoacetyltriglycine. *Radiology* 1989;170:721–725.

Chapter 7

Musculoskeletal System

Several pharmaceuticals have been used to study the soft tissues and bones of the musculoskeletal system. This chapter considers bone, marrow, and the soft tissues separately.

Bone

Most studies of bone metabolism are currently done with Tc-99m-methylene diphosphonate (Tc-99m-MDP). Following injection, metabolic images are obtained at approximately 2 hours (Fig. 7–1). At this time approximately one-third of the pharmaceutical has been excreted in the urine, one-third has been cleared by the bones, and one-third remains in the extracellular space. The uptake of bone tracers appears to depend on blood flow and on the amount of calcium-containing bone crystal in the tissue. Autoradiographic studies have suggested that the specific locations of increased uptake in metabolically active bone are new blood vessels, osteoclasts, and hydroxyapatite; one or more of these locations is involved in any process in which bone metabolism is increased (Table 7–1).

Focally increased uptake of bone tracers occurs in the normal skeleton at sites of high metabolism. These sites include the growth plates in children and the sacroiliac joints. Abnormal focal uptake is usually the result of tumor, either primary or secondary; trauma, including focal mechanical stress; or infection. Inflammation adjacent to the periosteum also causes focally increased uptake.

Bone scintigraphy is frequently done in patients with known **malignant tumors** (Fig. 7–2). Initial scintigraphy is positive for solitary or multiple metastases in 43% of patients known to have cancer. The corresponding figures for specific tumors are shown in Table 7–2. In patients with known malignant tumors who have pain but normal radiographs, approximately 30% will have positive scintigraphy resulting from bone metastasis. The utility of scintigraphy in patients with known primary tumors but without pain is controversial. Patients with primary

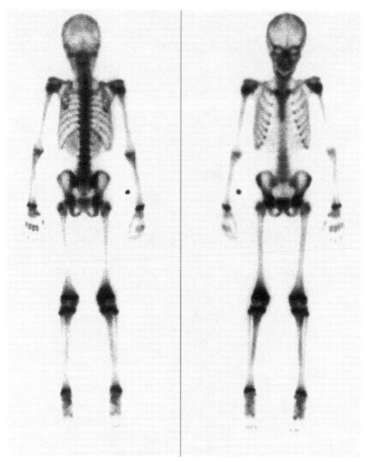

Figure 7–1. Normal bone Tc-99m-MDP study in an adolescent. Anterior (left) and posterior (right) views. Growth plates are active and therefore show high uptake of tracer. Other areas of relatively high uptake are the sacroiliac joint, midsacrum, and coracoid process.

tumors that frequently metastasize to bone (breast, prostate, and lung) may benefit from bone scintigraphy because pointless curative therapy may be avoided when metastases are discovered and because response to therapy can be monitored. This last issue is somewhat clouded by the flare phenomenon, in which the intensity and number of bone metastases appear to increase

Table 7–1.   Summary of Bone Scintigraphy Abnormalities

Focally increased uptake
  Trauma
    Fracture
    Ligamentous attachment injury
    Degenerative arthropathy
  Tumor
    Malignant
    Benign
  Infection
  Adjacent soft-tissue inflammation
    Arthritis
    Sinusitis
  Vascular
    Healing infarct or avascular necrosis
Focally decreased uptake
  Radiation therapy (remote)
  Tumor
    Rapidly growing
    Multiple myeloma
    Benign
  Vascular
    Infarct or avascular necrosis
    Increased intramedullary pressure
Diffusely increased uptake
    Widespread metastases
    Hyperparathyroidism
Diffuse apparently decreased uptake—increased soft-tissue uptake
  Renal failure
  Dermatomyositis

during the first few months after chemotherapy is instituted. The flare evidently results from increased bone metabolism resulting from healing rather than from progression of the metastases. Serial studies performed over a year or more may be necessary to distinguish flare from tumor progression. The flare phenomenon has been observed frequently in breast and prostate cancer and occurs in more than 90% of patients responding to therapy for breast cancer and in about 20% of nonresponders. A related phenomenon is focally increased uptake in the humeral heads, femoral heads, distal femurs, proximal tibias, sternum, and sacroiliac joints in patients receiving granulocyte colony stimulating factor.

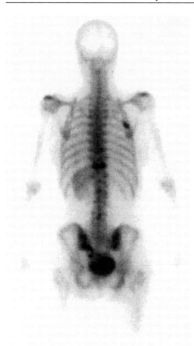

Figure 7–2.   Metastases. Foci of increased uptake in the right fourth rib, lower thoracic spine, lumbosacral spine, and left ilium represent metastases from renal adenocarcinoma. The right kidney has been removed.

TABLE 7–2.   Rates of Scintigraphy Positive for Bone Metastasis

Tumor	% Positive
Unknown primary	63
Breast	54
Multiple myeloma	54
Lung	53
Prostate	45
Head and neck	44
Miscellaneous	42
Gastrointestinal	41
Genitourinary (nonprostate, nongynecological, nontesticular)	37
Gynecological	29
Hodgkin's lymphoma	25
Lymphoma	10
Melanoma	10
Testicular	8

At the time of presentation, patients with known **breast cancer** have metastases detected on bone scintigraphy at rates of 2% at stage 2 and 35% at stage 3. It has been argued that patients with small localized primary breast carcinomas without clinical evidence for metastasis are so unlikely to have detectable bone metastases that bone scintigraphy is not indicated in this group. The corresponding figures for prostate cancer are 5% at stage 1, 10% at stage 2, and 20% at stage 3.

Radiographic correlation can be used to improve the specificity of bone scintigraphy. A lack of radiographic abnormality in regions of increased uptake increases the likelihood of tumor as the cause of increased uptake. However, **trauma** and **degenerative arthropathy** may also cause increased uptake without radiographic findings. In patients with known primary tumors, solitary lesions are encountered in about 15% of cases; 64% of these are due to metastasis. In this setting, radiographic correlation is important because of the possibility of detecting a benign cause of increased uptake.

The distribution of foci of bone uptake sometimes gives a clue as to the primary tumor. Early **prostate cancer** metastases tend to be in the pelvis and lumbar spine. **Leukemic deposits** and **lymphomas** are often seen near the ends of long bones (Fig. 7–3). Solitary foci near the organ of origin may represent direct extension (Fig. 7–4).

Nonmalignant focal bone growths—including **cysts, osteomas, eosinophilic granuloma, brown tumors, fibrous dysplasia,** and **Paget's disease**—often cause increased uptake (Figs. 7–5 through 7–9). Increased uptake can be detected scintigraphically even when roentgenograms are negative. Radionuclide bone imaging or a simple collimated probe can be used intraoperatively to localize and direct therapy of osteoid osteomas.

Trauma accounts for a significant percentage of the indications for bone scintigraphy and is a common cause of focally increased uptake (Fig. 7–, 10, 11). The accuracy of scintigraphy increases with increasing time following trauma. Ninety-five percent of patients under 65 years of age have positive scintigraphy within 24 hours of trauma, and a significant proportion is positive earlier than 24 hours. Ninety-five percent of fractures in patients of all ages are positive by 3 days; this figure rises to 98% at 1 week. When performed with modern equipment and diphosphonate tracers, scintigraphy is sufficiently accurate to be

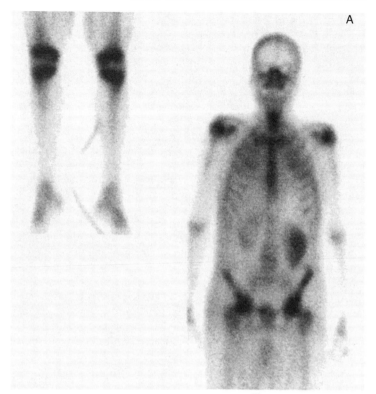

Figure 7–3. *continued*

performed at the time of presentation, even within hours of trauma. Equivocal or negative initial studies can be followed up on subsequent days if necessary. The overall sensitivity and specificity of scintigraphy in a group of adult patients of all ages studied at various times between 0 and 72 hours after trauma are greater than 90%.

Stress fractures result when the normal rate of replacement of stressed bone exceeds the rate of resorption. Mechanical stress causes an initial resorption of cortical bone followed by replacement with denser bone. During the initial resorption phase, continued stress may eventually lead to fracture. This mechanism explains fractures seen in athletes and military recruits, especially when untrained individuals engage in repeated exercise

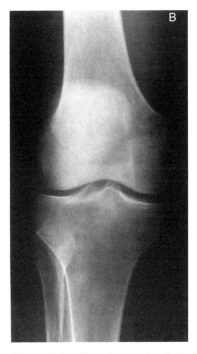

Figure 7–3. Chronic granulocytic leukemia. Increased uptake in the epiphyseal and adjacent metaphyseal regions of the femurs and tibias near the knee joints in **(A)** the anterior view of a Tc-99m-MDP bone study corresponds to **(B)** a permeative lytic pattern in the same regions on a roentgenogram of the right knee.

over a period of time. The fracture may appear after only hours of strenuous exercise in an untrained patient or after weeks or more of strenuous training in an experienced athlete. Stress fractures can occur in any bone but are most frequently seen in the tibia and fibula (Fig. 7–12). To evaluate the extent of a stress fracture accurately with scintigraphy, at least two views are required—typically, anterior and lateral. Complete stress fractures involve the entire circumference of a tubular bone rather than a focal segment of the circumference. Focal lesions that do not involve the entire circumference represent focal resorption from mechanical stress; these foci will become complete frac-

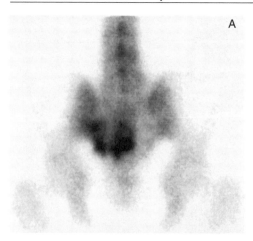

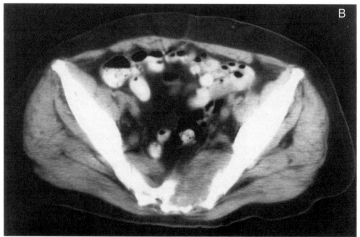

Figure 7–4.   Prostate carcinoma. **(A)** A posterior pelvic image from a Tc-99m-MDP bone study shows a region of increased uptake involving the left side of the sacrum and the left ilium. **(B)** A computed tomographic image through this region reveals prostate cancer extending from the adjacent soft tissues into the bone.

tures if the stress is continued. The differentiation of full cortex involvement from prefracture injuries is important because the earlier lesions can be treated with 1 or 2 weeks of avoidance the

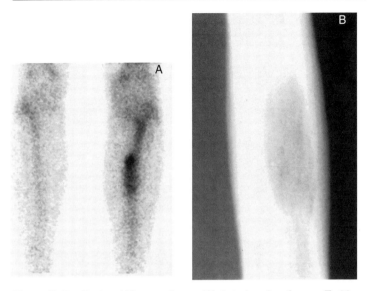

Figure 7–5. Eosinophilic granuloma. **(A)** Anterior view from a Tc-99m-MDP bone study shows a focus of increased uptake in the left tibia. **(B)** Roentgenogram shows a lytic focus.

stress, whereas complete fractures may require 6 weeks of complete rest. Rapid-sequence perfusion images may be acquired to determine the age of the stress fracture. Increased perfusion is seen in fractures less than several weeks old.

Repeated mechanical stress at the points of bony attachment of Sharpey's muscle fibers can result in focally increased uptake of bone tracers (see Fig. 7–12, 13). This phenomenon is seen in the legs of runners with **shin splints** and in other bones in which muscle attachments to bone are stressed. In the tibia, tracer uptake tends to be linearly distributed along a longer segment of bone than is seen in the uptake in a stress fracture. A second differential feature of shin splints is lack of increased perfusion in all stages of the injury.

Spondylolysis is probably a traumatic fracture of the pars interarticularis and may cause back pain. Abnormal scintigraphic activity at the site of spondylolysis has been correlated with pain, whereas pars defects without increased tracer uptake

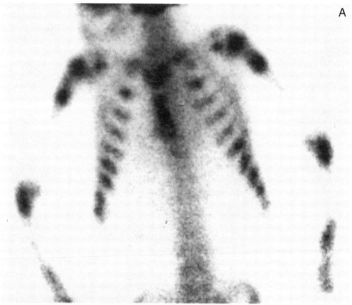

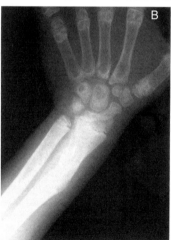

Figure 7–6. Hyperparathyroidism. **(A)** Anterior view of a Tc-99m-MDP bone study in a child with multiple brown tumors shows foci of increased uptake in the proximal humeral diaphyses and distal radial diaphyses. **(B)** Radiograph of the right wrist shows changes of hyperparathyroidism including a brown tumor in the distal radial diaphysis.

are more likely to be unassociated with pain. Single photon emission computed tomography (SPECT) imaging is more sensitive than planar imaging and is more accurate for precise localization of the abnormal uptake (Fig. 7–14).

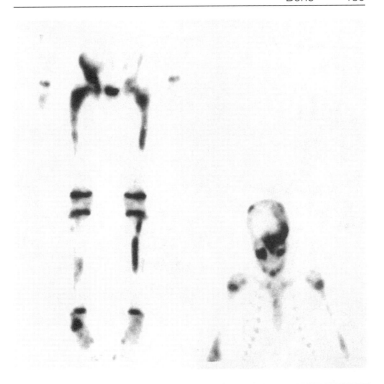

Figure 7–7. Polyostotic fibrous dysplasia. **(A)** Anterior view from a Tc-99m-MDP bone scan shows multiple foci of intensely increased uptake in the humeri, right ilium, right ischium, femurs, tibias, fibulas, right ankle, skull, and mandible. **(B)** Skull roentgenogram shows regions of sclerosis corresponding to the foci of increased bone tracer uptake.

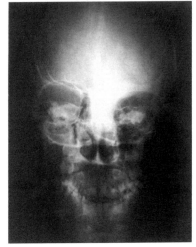

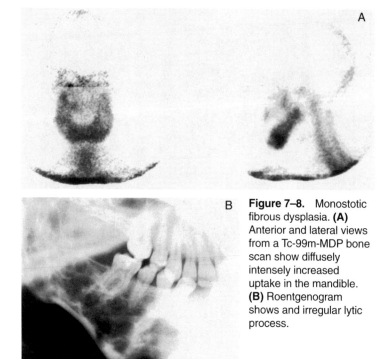

Figure 7–8. Monostotic fibrous dysplasia. **(A)** Anterior and lateral views from a Tc-99m-MDP bone scan show diffusely intensely increased uptake in the mandible. **(B)** Roentgenogram shows and irregular lytic process.

Trauma occasionally results in the **reflex sympathetic dystrophy** syndrome, a complex consisting of pain, tenderness, vasomotor instability, swelling, and dystrophic skin changes. Precipitating events other than trauma include certain drugs and neurologic abnormalities. A specific cause is never found in about one-third of cases. Commonly involved regions include the hands, wrists, knees, and ankles. Scintigraphy shows increased uptake on delayed images in the involved bones, especially in the periartic-ular regions. During the first 20 weeks from onset, increased perfusion and blood pool activity are seen on early images. Between 20 and 60 weeks, perfusion and blood pool images become normal, and between 60 and 100 weeks, delayed images become normal. In the 60- to 100-week interval, perfusion and blood pool images may show decreased radioactivity. The sensi-tivity of scintigraphy in the diagnosis of this condition is 62 to

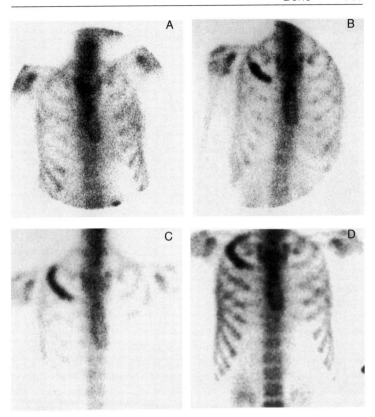

Figure 7–9. Paget's disease. Following a normal Tc-99m-MDP bone study **(A)**, successive studies done at 1-year intervals show Paget's disease of the right second rib starting at the distal end of the bone and progressing proximally **(B-D).**

96%, and the specificity is 92 to 97%. Early positivity appears to correlate with success of subsequent corticosteroid therapy.

Acute osteomyelitis is a cause of focal scintigraphic abnormality. The classic findings are focally increased uptake in rapid-sequence perfusion images, blood pool images, and delayed images (Fig. 7–15). The presence of these findings differentiates acute osteomyelitis from adjacent **cellulitis.** Pitfalls include **chronic osteomyelitis** in which the perfusion and blood pool

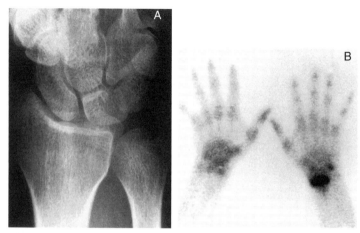

Figure 7–10. Radial fracture. **(A)** In a patient with a high clinical suspicion for distal radial fracture the roentgenogram was negative. **(B)** Delayed palmer views from a Tc-99m-MDP bone scan show intensely increased uptake in the right distal radius corresponding to a nondisplaced fracture.

images may not show increased activity; vascular tumors and fractures, which may have findings identical to the findings of acute osteomyelitis; and involvement of small bones in the hands and feet. If the affected bone is too small to distinguish from the adjacent soft tissues, the determination of whether increased perfusion or blood pool radioactivity is in the bone or the soft tissues may be impossible. In such a situation cellulitis overlying a noninfectious focal abnormality in a small bone may be misinterpreted scintigraphically as acute osteomyelitis. In addition, soft-tissue inflammation immediately adjacent to bone can cause increased bone uptake of tracer even when the bone is not infected (Fig. 7–16).

The differentiation of **osteomyelitis** from **vascular tumors, diabetic arthropathy,** or noninfected **fracture** may be impossible with Tc-99m-MDP. Such a differentiation may be accomplished with follow-up imaging with Ga-67, In-111 WBCs, Tc-99m-HMPAO WBCs (Fig. 7–17), or In-111 IgG. Ga-67 imaging is complicated by the uptake of gallium in noninfectious bone lesions. For this reason Ga-67 uptake in the region in question must be compared with Tc-99m-MDP uptake in the same

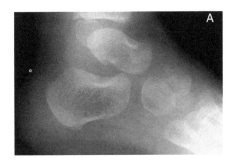

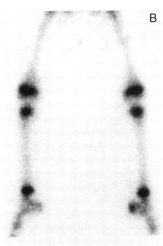

Figure 7–11. Battered child syndrome. **(A)** Roentgenogram of the right ankle in a child with unexplained trauma fails to demonstrate a fracture. **(B)** Focally increased uptake in the left calcaneus in an anterior view from a Tc-99m-MDP bone scan is highly suggestive of an occult fracture. **(C)** T1-weighted magnetic resonance imaging through the left calcaneus shows a low-signal region corresponding to the fracture. Bone scanning is useful in cases of suspected child abuse because of its ability to demonstrate multiple fractures and foci of periosteal trauma of various ages.

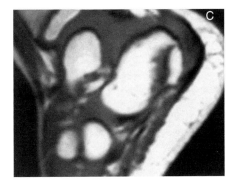

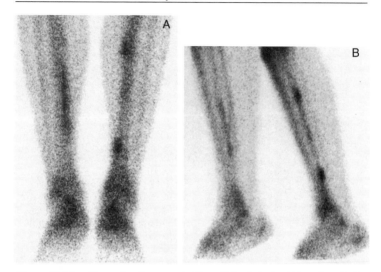

Figure 7–12. Stress fractures and shin splints. Anterior **(A)** and posterior **(B)** Tc-99m-MDP bone scan images show focal noncircumferential foci of increased uptake in the right proximal and distal tibia indicative of incomplete stress fractures. The linear regions of increased uptake in both tibias represent shin splints.

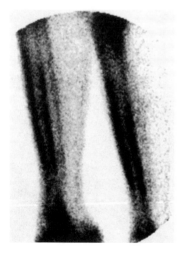

Figure 7–13. Shin splints. Lateral views from a Tc-99m-MDP bone study in a 21-year-old runner show regions of intensely increased uptake along muscle attachments to the tibias. Focal uptake suggestive of stress fracture is not apparent.

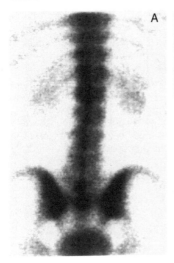

Figure 7–14. Pars interarticularous defect. This 28-year-old javelin thrower with low back pain and a known L5 left pars interarticularous defect had a negative Tc-99m-MDP bone study (**A,** posterior view). (**B**) Two levels from a transaxial SPECT bone study show increased uptake in the region of the left pars interarticularous, suggesting that the pain is associated with the defect.

region. More intense Ga-67 uptake than Tc-99m-MDP uptake suggests infection. The sensitivity and specificity of this approach are in the 60 to 80% range. The sensitivity and specificity of In-111-WBC imaging for osteomyelitis are 80 to 95%; however, not all reports have been this favorable. Causes of false-positive In-111-WBC imaging are aseptic chronic inflammation, loosening of prostheses, rheumatoid arthritis, and some tumors. The sensitivity of imaging with Tc-99m-MDP, Ga-67, and In-111 WBCs is greater in acute than in chronic infection.

Nonspecific polyclonal human IgG labeled with In-111 has recently been shown to be sensitive in the detection of musculoskeletal inflammation, including acute and chronic infection and sterile inflammatory prosthesis. In this procedure injection of 75 MBq of In-111 IgG is followed by static images at 4, 24, and 48 hours. A positive study is indicated by increasing accumulation of tracer over time.

The evaluation of **knee and hip prostheses** can be carried out with Tc-99m-MDP. Mild diffuse increased uptake around the prosthesis is often seen as much as several years after surgery. Focal increased uptake at the tip of the femoral component of a cemented hip prosthesis 1 year after surgery strongly suggests loosening (Fig. 7–18). Intense uptake around a prosthesis suggests infection, and this situation can be further clarified with

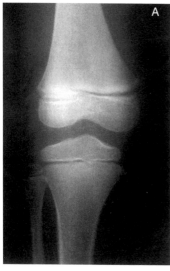

Figure 7–15. Osteomyelitis. A 12-year-old male had knee pain and a normal roentgenogram **(A).** Perfusion **(B),** immediate static **(C),** and 2-hour delayed **(D)** anterior views of a Tc99m-MDP bone study show increased tracer. This combination of scintigraphic findings is typical of osteomyelitis but is also seen in vascular tumors, some fractures, and diabetic arthropathy.

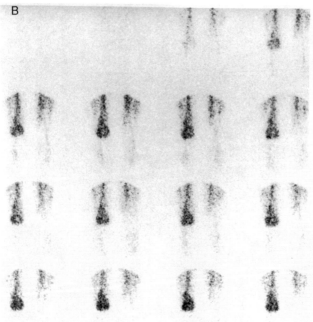

Figure 7–15. *continued*

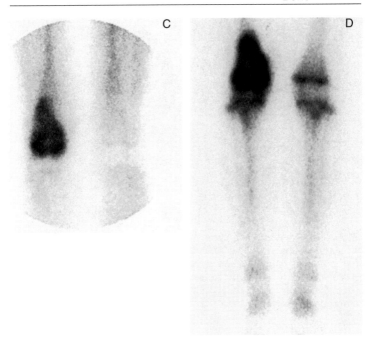

three-phase Tc-99m-MDP imaging (Fig. 7–19) or with gallium, In-111 WBCs, Tc-99m-HMPAO WBCs, or In-111 IgG.

Increased Tc-99m-MDP uptake is seen in essentially all the **arthritides.** Although bone imaging is not generally used to diagnose arthritis, this condition must be kept in mind when positive bone image findings are being evaluated. **Septic arthritis** results in increased perfusion and blood pool activity in the region of the joint. Uptake in the bones of an infected joint is frequently increased because of irritation of the bone surface by the adjacent inflammation. When the infection extends into the bone with resultant frank osteomyelitis, the intensity of tracer uptake increases, and the uptake extends deeper into the bone (Fig. 7–20). All three phases of the Tc-99m-MDP bone study are typically positive in **diabetic arthropathy** (Fig. 7–21. Patients at risk for this condition are frequently also at risk for osteomyelitis in the same regions, and labeled WBC imaging may be necessary to differentiate infection from arthropathy. The sensitivity of the combination of Tc-99m-MDP scintigraphy and In-111-WBC scintigraphy in this situation is close to 100%, and the speci-

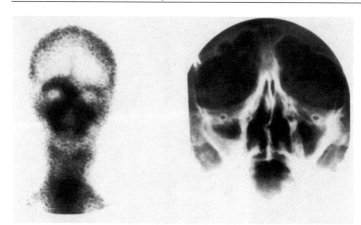

Figure 7–16. Acute and chronic sinusitis. Anterior view of skull from a Tc-99m-MDP bone study (left) shows increased uptake of tracer in bones that are adjacent to inflamed mucosa. These bones are not infected but are reacting to adjacent inflammation in the paranasal sinuses. Roentgenogram (right) shows changes of sinusitis in the maxillary antra, ethmoid sinuses, and right frontal sinus.

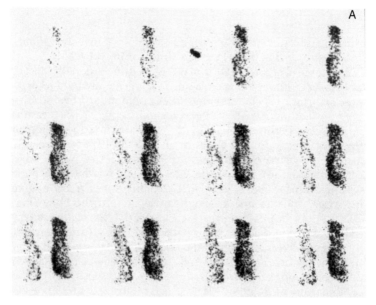

Figure 7–16. *continued*

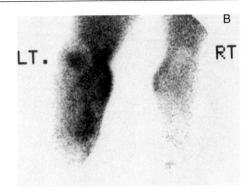

Figure 7–17. Osteomyelitis. Anterior perfusion images **(A)** from at Tc-99m-MDP bone study show diffusely increased perfusion of the medial aspect of the left foot and ankle corresponding to a region of soft-tissue erythema and underlying diabetic arthropathy of the foot and ankle. Increased uptake is seen in a similar distribution in plantar immediate static **(B)** and delayed **(C)** views. These findings may reflect diabetic arthropathy, infection, or both. **(D)** A plantar view done 3 hours after injection of Tc-99m-HMPAO-WBCs shows a focus of increased uptake in the distal end of the left first metatarsal, which proved to represent osteomyelitis.

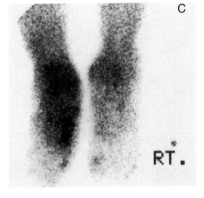

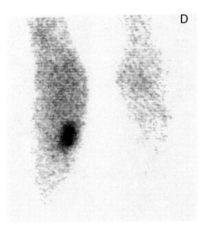

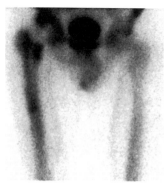

Figure 7–18. Loose hip prosthesis. Increased tracer uptake in a Tc-99m-MDP bone study around the proximal end of the femoral component and focally at the distal end of the femoral component several years after surgery suggests loosening. Increased uptake around the acetabular component is also suggestive of loosening. A normal perfusion study militated against infection.

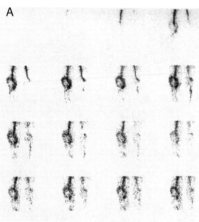

Figure 7–19. Infected knee prosthesis. Increased intensity in the perfusion **(A),** immediate static **(B),** and delayed **(C)** anterior images from a Tc-99m-MDP bone study adjacent to the tibial and femoral components of the left knee prosthesis in this patient with bilateral knee prosthesis suggests infection.

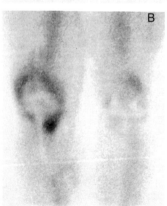

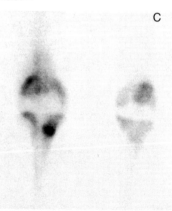

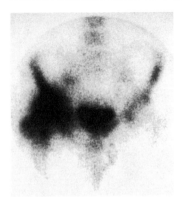 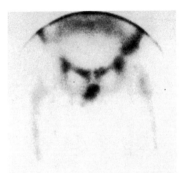

Figure 7–20. **(A)** Septic hip. Anterior view of the pelvis from a Tc-99m-MDP bone study shows intensely increased uptake in the right proximal femur and acetabulum. Pus was aspirated from the right hip. Although infected joint fluid may cause increased uptake of bone tracer by bones adjacent to the fluid without actual osteomyelitis, the degree of bone uptake in this case is suggestive of osteomyelitis. **(B)** A corresponding Tc-99m-sulfur colloid study shows decreased uptake in the right proximal femur and right acetabulum caused either by destruction of marrow resulting from infection or by decreased blood supply to the marrow secondary to high intramedullary pressures caused by intramedullary infection. The femur and acetabulum proved in this case to be infected.

ficity is about 83%. **Osteoarthritis** frequently causes focal increased Tc-99m-MDP uptake. The intensity of uptake varies from mild to intense. Perfusion and blood pool images are typically normal.

Osteonecrosis (avascular necrosis) is characterized by intense uptake of tracer adjacent to the infarcted region. In some cases the infarcted bone can be seen as a photon-deficient area (Fig. 7–22. Scintigraphy is an accurate method to diagnose Legg-Calve-Perthes disease, which is characterized initially by a photon-deficient region followed by increased uptake in reactive bone over the ensuing months.

Diffusely increased uptake in the skeleton is characterized by apparently reduced activity in the soft tissues and in the urinary tract when images are properly exposed for the bones. Commonly encountered causes of the "super scan" are **renal osteodystrophy** and **diffuse metastases** from primary tumors of the

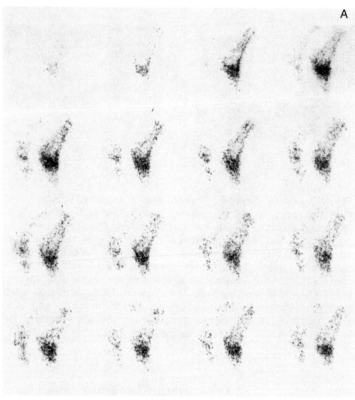

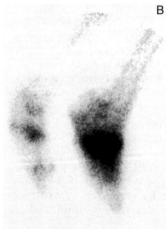

Figure 7–21. *continued*

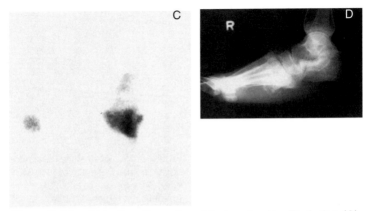

Figure 7–21. Diabetic arthropathy of foot and ankle. Perfusion **(A),** immediate static **(B),** and delayed **(C)** images from a Tc-99m-MDP bone study. View of the right foot and ankle is lateral and that of the left foot and ankle is medial. **(D)** Roentgenogram shows findings typical of diabetic arthropathy of the ankle. Increased tracer activity on all three phases of the bone study is typical of either diabetic arthropathy or infection, and an additional study, such as a Tc-99m-WBC study, would be necessary to differentiate between these two possibilities.

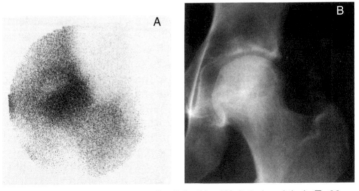

Figure 7–22. Avascular necrosis of the hip. **(A)** Anterior pinhole Tc-99m-MDP image of the left hip shows a subcortical photon-deficient region corresponding to a necrotic focus. Immediately distal to the photon-deficient region is a band of increased tracer uptake corresponding to reparative bone. **(B)** Corresponding roentgenogram shows a subcortical fracture and mixed lysis and sclerosis in the femoral head.

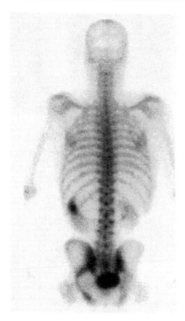

Figure 7–23. Metastatic renal adenocarcinoma. Posterior Tc-99m-MDP study shows a large, relatively photon-deficient region in the left side of the pelvis centered at the acetabulum. This region corresponds to a metastasis and is surrounded by a rim of increased tracer uptake in reactive bone around the tumor. The upper pole of the left kidney is distorted and displaced laterally by the primary tumor.

prostate, lung, and breast. **Primary hyperparathyroidism** occasionally results in diffusely increased bone tracer uptake.

As discussed earlier, **focally decreased bone tracer uptake** occurs in **bone infarcts.** Other causes include **tumors** and focal **radiation therapy. Multiple myeloma** and focal **plasmacytomas** frequently cause focal defects, but bone imaging may be normal (66% of cases) or show focally increased uptake in these conditions. Other tumors that may cause focal photon-deficient bone lesions are **bronchogenic carcinoma** and **breast cancer.** When caused by carcinoma metastases, photon-deficient lesions suggest rapid tumor growth. These lesions may appear as pure defects or as photon-deficient defects surrounded by increased uptake (Fig. 7–23). Photon-deficient focal lesions are usually seen as lytic radiographic defects; however, lytic radiographic defects associated with tumors are usually associated with focally increased bone tracer uptake. Diffusely decreased skeletal uptake has not been reliably correlated with pathologic conditions and is most likely a normal variant. In particular, this finding is not a reliable indicator of osteoporosis.

Marrow

Two methods of marrow imaging have been used. In the first, radioactive iron is administered. The iron becomes bound to transferrin and is incorporated into erythroid precursors. In the second, more common approach, a radioactive colloid, usually Tc-99m-sulfur colloid, is administered and becomes phagocytized by the reticuloendothelial system. Because this second approach is simpler and less expensive than the first and because abnormalities in the erythron and the reticuloendothelial system tend to parallel each other, Tc-99m-sulfur colloid is usually used for marrow imaging. Marrow abnormalities are manifested as focally or diffusely decreased uptake of Tc-99m-sulfur colloid. The main uses of marrow imaging are the detection of **osteonecrosis,** the detection and localization of **metastases,** and the evaluation of the marrow's **response to radiation and chemotherapy.** Marrow imaging is positive in about 83% of **multiple myeloma** cases.

In the evaluation of avascular necrosis of the hip (Fig. 7–24), the accuracy of Tc-99m-sulfur colloid imaging has been reported to be as high as 95%, but only when there is adequate red marrow in the hips for evaluation. Essentially all patients below 20 years of age show marrow uptake in the femoral heads, but this figure is only 37% for subjects aged 70 to 79. Marrow imaging is also useful in the detection of **infarcts** in

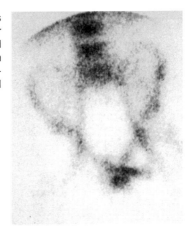

Figure 7–24. Avascular necrosis of the right proximal femur. Anterior view from a Tc-99m-sulfur colloid study shows absent tracer uptake in the right proximal femur, corresponding to a necrotic femoral head.

patients with **sickle cell disease.** This study can be used to differentiate infarcts from other causes of pain. More than half of patients with sickle cell disease undergoing marrow imaging show painless marrow infarcts, so serial imaging may be required to differentiate new from old infarcts. Cortical bone infarcts tend to be very painful, are associated with marrow imaging defects, and often change from initially cold to hot within days on Tc-99m-MDP bone imaging.

Extramedullary hematopoiesis occasionally occurs as a solid tumor outside of the liver or spleen. Imaging with Tc-99m-sulfur colloid distinguishes these lesions from other solid tumors. The technique is not useful for tumors in the liver and spleen because of the high degree of normal colloid uptake in these organs.

The general status of the marrow can be evaluated in patients undergoing marrow obliteration in preparation for **bone marrow transplant** and in patients with **myelofibrosis** and **aplastic anemia;** no colloid uptake is seen in these conditions. With successful treatment, repopulation of the marrow results in reappearance of colloid uptake.

Soft Tissues

Tc-99m-MDP accumulates in soft tissues when they contain an excess of calcium. Soft-tissue calcium excess tends to occur locally in **necrotic or ischemic lesions** (Fig. 7–25) or more diffusely in **hyperparathyroidism** (Fig. 7–26). **Strokes** and **myocardial infarctions** are occasionally seen on bone scans. Breast uptake of bone-seeking agents is commonly seen; this finding is nonspecific and occurs in benign and malignant diseases as well as in normal breasts.

Increased uptake is seen in skeletal muscle undergoing **rhabdomyolysis.** Rhabdomyolysis may occur following trauma, including **exercise, electrical burns** (Fig. 7–27), **frostbite,** and **intramuscular injections,** or in **alcohol abuse.** Muscle uptake is also seen in calcifying muscle diseases such as **polymyositis, dermatomyositis** (Fig. 7–28), **scleroderma,** and **myositis ossificans.**

Gastrointestinal uptake can be the result of **necrotizing enterocolitis** in infants or ischemic bowel in adults; Tc-99m-MDP imaging may be diagnostically useful in these conditions. The stomach and lungs are common sites of increased tracer accumulation in patients with **hypercalcemia** (Fig. 7–26).

Figure 7–25. Necrotic liver. Anterior Tc-99m-MDP study shows intense uptake in a massively necrotic liver. This 44-year-old woman had extension of a primary renal carcinoma into the superior vena cava and hepatic veins with subsequent hepatic necrosis. Sufficient hepatic blood flow persisted for delivery of tracer to the necrotic tissue. There are metastases in the right femur.

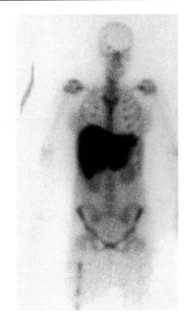

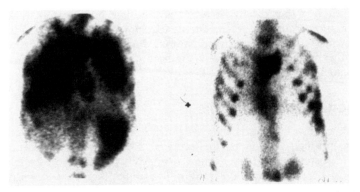

Figure 7–26. Soft-tissue uptake in a patient with hypercalcemia. A 66-year-old woman with breast cancer had hypercalcemia as part of a paraneoplastic syndrome. Initial anterior Tc-99m-MDP bone study (left) shows intense tracer uptake in the lungs and stomach, a pattern typical of hypercalcemia. Six months following chemotherapy and resolution of hypercalcemia lung and stomach uptake have disappeared (right); multiple foci of increased uptake at sites of bone metastasis persist.

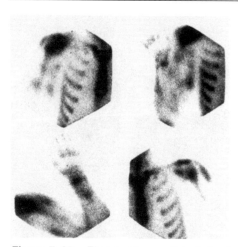

Figure 7–27. Electrical burns. Selected anterior views from a Tc-99m-MDP study show multiple foci of increased uptake in the soft tissues of the upper extremities. These foci represent tissue necrosis secondary to electrical burns sustained in an accident by this lineman.

Tumors that calcify or ossify accumulate bone tracers. The common examples are **mucinous carcinomas** of the ovary and colon (Fig. 7–29), **neuroblastoma,** and **osteosarcoma.** Bone tracer is sometimes seen in **malignant pleural effusions** and **malignant ascites** (Fig. 7–30).

Bone Mineral Analysis

Bone density measurements are potentially important because of the morbidity and mortality that result from fractures in patients with **osteoporosis.** Bone mineral appears to decrease through most of adult life, more rapidly in women, and most rapidly after menopause. Bone loss can also be caused by **Cushing's disease, thyrotoxicosis, anorexia nervosa, tamoxifen,** and **hypoparathyroidism.** Bone mineral analysis has been proposed as a method to detect osteoporosis, monitor the results of its therapy, determine fracture risk, and monitor skeletal effects of drugs that cause osteoporosis. Of fractures occurring in osteoporosis, those of the hip and lumbar spine are the most expen-

Figure 7–28. Dermatomyositis. Anterior view from a Tc-99m-MDP bone study shows multiple regions of tracer uptake in calcified skeletal muscles.

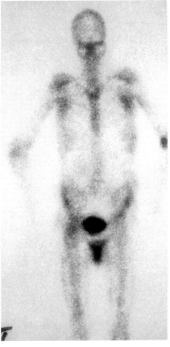

sive and result in greatest mortality and morbidity, so these regions receive most clinical attention.

In single-energy absorptiometry a monoenergetic source, typically I-125, is placed on one side of the body part to be analyzed, and a detector is placed on the other side. This method gives reasonable results for bones such as the distal radius and the calcaneus, which are not surrounded by much soft tissue. Calculation of bone density requires an assumption regarding the attenuation resulting from soft tissues, so bones deep in the body such as the proximal femur and lumbar spine cannot be reliably evaluated with this method.

In dual-energy absorptiometry a source such as Gd-153, which has energy peaks at about 44 and 100 keV, is used with a detection system having two energy windows. The absorption effects of soft tissue and bone can be determined independently by solving a system of two equations (one for each energy) and two unknowns (the absorptions of soft tissue and bone). The

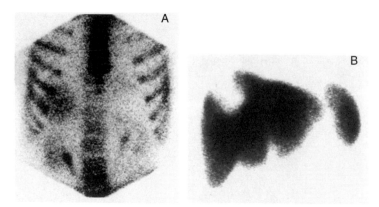

Figure 7–29. Colon carcinoma metastatic to liver. **(A)** Anterior Tc-99m-MDP view shows a large region of increased uptake projecting over the liver in this patient with known mucinous carcinoma of the colon. Anterior view from a Tc-99m-sulfur colloid study **(B)** shows a focal defect corresponding to the metastasis.

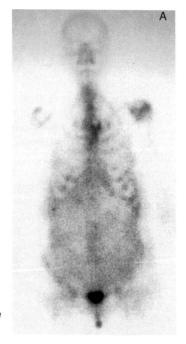

Figure 7–30. *continued*

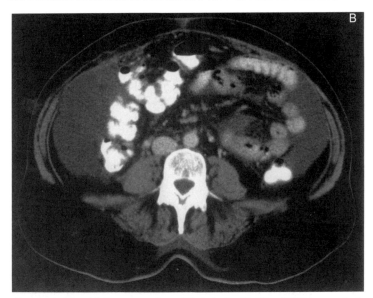

Figure 7–30. Malignant ascites. **(A)** Anterior Tc-99m-MDP bone study shows diffusely increased uptake in the abdomen of this 65-year-old woman with breast cancer and ascites. **(B)** A CT study confirmed the ascites. Bone tracer uptake is also sometimes seen in plural effusions.

source is narrowly collimated and scans the body part of interest, yielding a transmission image along with the quantitative data. This image is used to detect the presence of compression fractures or degenerative changes that would result in erroneous bone mineral calculations. Local tissues receive very low radiation doses, usually about 5 to 15 mrad.

The methods of bone mineral analysis are characterized by measures of precision and reliability. Precision is a measure of test reproducibility. A highly precise test would have a low percentage of variability when the same measurement is made repeatedly. Reliability is a measure of a correlation of the test result with a gold standard. A highly reliable test for bone mineral would have a low-percentage variation from the known mineral content of a phantom. Dual-energy absorptiometry has a precision of 1 to 3% and a reliability of 4 to 6%.

Radionuclide Therapy of Painful Bone Lesions

Several agents have been used to treat painful skeletal foci that have increased uptake of these agents. P-32 and Sr-89 in their ionic forms are taken up by osteoblastic bone lesions. Other nuclides are chelated to ligands that accumulate in focal bone lesions. Examples are RE-186-HEDP and SM-153-EDTMP. The mode of action of all these agents is destruction of tumor cells by local beta radiation. Improvement in pain is frequently preceded by a flare in symptoms that lasts for several days following therapy. Pain relief is temporary, lasting several months on the average. Therapy can be repeated with reduced efficacy in each successive treatment. The major complication is bone marrow depression.

Most of the studies involving these agents have not been blind. Patients in the studies have remained on pain medications, and in some cases hormone therapy was used with nuclide therapy. The quoted percentages of patients responding may be exaggerations of the efficacy of this form of therapy. There is no evidence that life is prolonged.

P-32 in its orthophosphate form has been used to treat metastases since the 1940s. This nuclide is produced in a cyclotron and liberates beta particles of 1.71 MeV energy. The half-life is 14.3 days. Five to 20 mCi intravenous doses are frequently given with androgen or parathyroid hormone treatment to enhance uptake in metastases. About 84% of **breast cancer** patients and 77% of **prostate cancer** patients respond.

Sr-89 is reactor-produced. This nuclide liberates 1.43-MeV beta particles and has a half-life of 50.5 days. Doses near 40 μCi/kg have response rates very similar to those for P-32.

RE-186 has been used in a form chelated to a diphosphonate ligand (RE-186-HEDP). RE-186 has a 90-hour half-life. Beta particles of 1.07 MeV energy are liberated along with 137–keV gamma particles. The gamma radiation allows imaging, evaluation of uptake, quantitative radiation dosimetry, and dose calculation. The response rate was 77% in a blind crossover study involving mostly **prostate and breast cancers.** The recommended dose is 30 to 35 mCi.

SM-153-EDTMP, another chelate, has recently undergone preliminary testing. SM-153 is reactor-produced and has a half-life of 46 hours. Beta particles are liberated with energies of 640, 710, and 810 keV. One hundred-three-keV gamma radiation allows for imaging and radiation dosimetry. The optimum administered dosage appears to be 0.75 to 1.0 mCi/kg. In a study involving somewhat lower administered doses, the response rate was 65%.

Suggested Readings

Campa JA, Payne R: The management of intractable bone pain: A clinician's perspective. *Semin Nucl Med* 1992;22:3-10.

Coleman RE, Mashiter G, Whitaker KB, Moss DW, Rubens RD, Fogelman I: Bone scan flare predicts successful systemic therapy for bone metastases. *J Nucl Med* 1988;29:1354-1359.

Coleman RE, Rubens RD, Fogelman I: Reappraisal of the baseline bone scan in breast cancer. *J Nucl Med* 1988;29:1045-1049.

Collier BD, Johnson RP, Carrera GF, et al: Painful spondylosis or spondylolisthesis studied by radiography and single-photon emission computed tomography. *Radiology* 1985;154:207–211.

Corcoran RJ, Thrall JH, Kyle RW, Kaminski RJ, Johnson MC: *Radiology* 1976;121:663-667.

Datz FL, Taylor A Jr: The clinical use of radionuclide bone marrow imaging. *Semin Nucl Med* 1985;15:239.

Demangeat JL, Constantinesco A, Brunot B, Foucher G, Farcot JM: Three-phase bone scanning in reflex sympathetic dystrophy of the hand. *J Nucl Med* 1988;29:26-32.

Fogelman I: An evaluation of the contribution of bone mass measurements to clinical practice. *Semin Nucl Med* 1989;19:62-68.

Front D, Israel O: Nuclear medicine in monitoring response to cancer treatment. *J Nucl Med* 1989;10:1731-1736.

Gentili A, Miron SD, Bellon EM: Nonosseous accumulation of bone-neck radiopharmaceuticals. *Radiographics* 1990;10:871-881.

Health and Public Policy Committee: Radiologic methods to evaluate bone mineral content. *Ann Int Med* 1984;100:908-911.

Holder LE: Clinical radionuclide bone imaging. *Radiology* 1990; 176:607–614.

Holder LE, Mackinnon SE: Reflex sympathetic dystrophy in the hands: clinical and scintigraphic criteria. *Radiology* 1984;152:517–522.

Holder LE, Schwartz C, Wernicke PG, Michael RH: Radionuclide bone imaging in the early detection of fractures of the proximal femur (hip): multifactorial analysis. *Radiology* 1990;174:509-515.

Kober B, Hermann HJ, Wetzel E: "Cold lesions" in bone scintigraphy. *Fortschr Röntgenstr* 1979;131:545-549.

Kozin F, Soin JS, Ryan LM, Carrera G, Wortmann RL: Bone scintigraphy in the reflux sympathetic dystrophy syndrome. *Radiology* 1981;138:437–443.

Lisbona R, Rosenthall L: Role of radionuclide imaging in osteoid osteoma. *AJR* 1979;132:77–80.

Matin P: Basic principles of nuclear medicine techniques for detection of evaluation of trauma and sports medicine injuries. *Semin Nucl Med* 1988;18:90-112.

Maxon HR III, Schroder LE, Hertzberg VS, et al: Rhenium-186(Sn)HEDP for treatment of painful osseous metastases: results of a double-blind crossover comparison with placebo. *J Nucl Med* 1991;32:1877–1881.

McAfee JG: What is the best method for imaging focal infections? *J Nucl Med* 1990;31:413-416. Editorial.

Pollen JJ, Witztum KF, Ashburn WL: The flare phenomenon on radionuclide bone scan in metastatic prostate cancer. *AJR* 1984;142:773-776.

Schauwecker DS: Osteomyelitis: diagnosis with In-111-labeled leukocytes. *Radiology* 1989;171:141-146.

Schauwecker DS, Park HM, Burt RW, Mock BH, Wellman HN: Combined bone scintigraphy and indium-111 leukocyte scans in neuropathic foot disease. *J Nucl Med* 1988;29:1651-1655.

Sy WM, Patel D, Faunce H: Significance of absent or faint kidney sign on bone scan. *J Nucl Med* 1975;16:454-456.

Tawn DJ, O'Hare JP, O'Brien AD, et al: Bone scintigraphy and radiography in the early recognition of diabetic osteopathy. *Br J Radiol* 1988;61:273-279.

Wahner HW, Dunn WL, Riggs BL: Assessment of Bone Mineral. Part 2. *J Nucl Med* 1984;25:1241-1253.

Chapter 8

Central Nervous System

The major radiopharmaceuticals currently used to image the brain are Tc-99m-DTPA and Tc-99m-HMPAO. Tc-99m-DTPA has been used for many years to image tumors and strokes; these lesions cause breakdown of the blood-brain barrier, allowing DTPA to enter the damaged tissue. Tc-99m-HMPAO is a fat-soluble pharmaceutical that crosses the blood–brain barrier, where it undergoes a chemical change that precludes its return to the vascular space. Tc-99m-HMPAO becomes distributed in the brain tissue in proportion to local blood flow; this tracer is usually used in conjunction with single photon emission computed tomography (SPECT) imaging to evaluate regional aberrations in blood flow that occur in such conditions as Alzheimer's disease, AIDS, and drug abuse.

Vascular Lesions

Strokes have traditionally been imaged with Tc-99m-labeled agents such as DTPA, pertechnetate, and glucoheptonate. Twenty mCi are injected as a bolus into a systemic vein. Serial 2- or 3-second images are obtained for 1 minute. Two- to 3-hour 500,000-count static images are obtained in the anterior, posterior, and lateral views. Strokes are characterized by decreased perfusion in the region of the stroke early in the flow study but by increased radioactivity in the same region later in the flow study ("flip-flop" phenomenon). The initial decrease in radioactivity in the region of the stroke reflects decreased perfusion secondary to the arterial occlusion. The later by increase in radioactivity in the flow study reflects hyperemia ("luxury perfusion") adjacent to the stroke. By 3 hours after injection, much of the radiopharmaceutical, especially in the case of Tc-99m-DTPA and Tc-99m-glucoheptonate, has been removed from the extracellular space by the kidneys. The pharmaceutical that has crossed the blood–brain barrier remains at the site of damage, creating a focus of increased intensity. These classic findings of

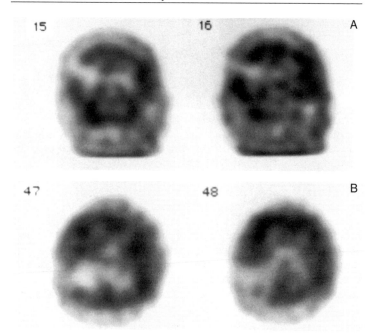

Figure 8-1. Cerebral ischemia. Coronal **(A)** and axial **(B)** slices selected from a Tc-99m-HMPAO study show decreased perfusion in the right parietal cerebral cortex. This patient had occlusion of the right internal carotid artery but no stroke.

stroke are reliably detected starting at about 2 days after the stroke, and they resolve over the ensuing weeks.

Asymmetry in the perfusion phase of the study in the face of normal delayed images is seen in **stenosis of the internal carotid artery** on the side showing less perfusion. Cerebral vascular disease can also be detected with SPECT imaging in conjunction with Tc-99m-HMPAO, as this agent becomes deposited in the brain in concentrations proportional to local blood flow. Imaging done between 20 minutes and several hours after injection will thus show decreased uptake in regions of **ischemia** (Fig. 8-1) or **infarction**. Although planar imaging can be performed, SPECT imaging increases the utility of the examination in localizing the ischemic region.

BRAIN DEATH

Brain death is associated with cerebral edema with resulting increased intracranial pressure that exceeds systolic blood pressure. This reduces cerebral blood flow to zero. Tc-99m-labeled radiopharmaceuticals such as Tc-99m-DTPA or Tc-99m-pertechnetate can be used to perform a perfusion study of the head and neck. In a positive study (one indicating brain death), rapid-sequence perfusion images show flow in the common carotid arteries and in the soft tissues exterior to the cranium. No flow is seen in the brain. The superior sagittal sinus is typically not visualized within the first minute after injection but may be seen faintly 5 to 10 minutes later (Figs. 8-2, 8-3). In a negative study the anterior and middle cerebral artery groups as well as the superior sagittal sinus are seen in the anterior projection during a 1 minute series of rapid-sequence serial images (Fig. 8-4). The test is highly specific in the sense that patients with a positive test essentially never survive. However, a negative test does not preclude impending brain death.

The quality of the radionuclide cerebral angiogram is somewhat dependent on the administration of a rapid intravenous bolus, which may not always be possible. This difficulty is avoided when Tc-99m-HMPAO is used. In this approach, 20 mCi of Tc-99m-HMPAO are administered intravenously. Five to 15 minutes after injection, anterior and both lateral views of the head are acquired. A positive study is indicated by absence of brain uptake of HMPAO.

Tumors

Computed tomography is somewhat more sensitive than scintigraphy in the detection of most tumors. However, the sensitivities of computed tomography (CT) and scintigraphy are similar for meningiomas and high-grade gliomas, and some of these tumors are detected with scintigraphy but not CT. The preferred imaging agent is Tc-99m-DTPA. Early-perfusion images may show increased radioactivity in vascular tumors. For example, **meningiomas** characteristically produce an early vascular blush that fades only minimally during the perfusion portion of the study. Delayed (2 to 3 hours) images show increased uptake in the brain tissue that has been damaged by a tumor. Tumors often

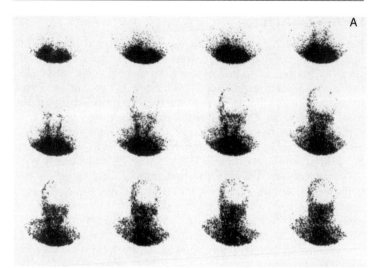

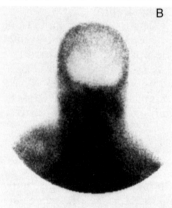

Figure 8-2. Brain death in an adult. Anterior 2-second perfusion images **(A)** and an immediate static image **(B)** show perfusion of the scalp and other structures supplied by the external carotid arteries but no radioactivity in the brain.

appear spherical, although a central region of decreased uptake may be seen in large tumors.

SPECT imaging with Tc-99m-HMPAO has not proved to be of significant value in the evaluation of most brain tumors, because the uptake of Tc-99m-HMPAO by tumors is variable. SPECT imaging following the administration of Tl-201 can be used to distinguish low- from high-grade **gliomas** and **lymphomas** from **infections** (Figs. 8-5, 8-6). The thallium uptake is

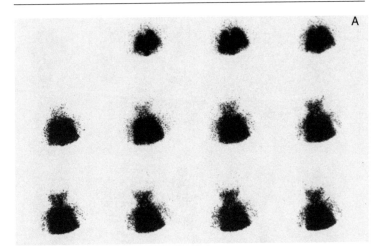

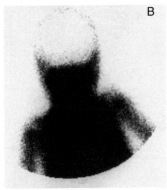

Figure 8-3. Brain death in an infant. Two-second anterior perfusion images **(A)** and an immediate anterior static image **(B)** following the administration of Tc-99m-DTPA failed to show brain radioactivity.

increased above normal brain tissue levels by a factor of about 1.3 in low-grade astrocytomas and 2.4 in high-grade tumors. Uptake is increased in lymphomas but not in infections. The accuracy of this test approaches 90%. Tl-201 SPECT offers the possibility of differentiating recurrent tumor from **scar** and **postsurgical changes.**

PET imaging is useful for detecting whether focal brain lesions are active tumor or posttherapeutic scar. F-18-fluorodeoxyglucose concentrate in metabolically active tissue such as tumor but to a lesser degree in scar tissue (Fig. 8-7).

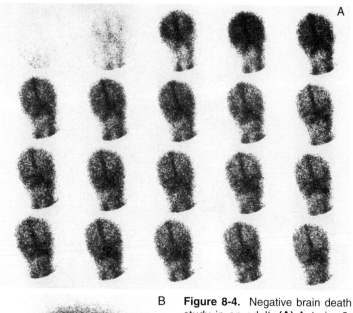

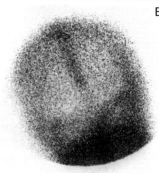

Figure 8-4. Negative brain death study in an adult. **(A)** Anterior 2-second perfusion images show the middle and anterior cerebral artery groups in early frames. The superior sagittal sinus is clearly visualized. Radioactivity in the brain is higher than that in the scalp. Anterior immediate static view **(B)** shows relatively intense radioactivity in the venous sinuses.

Dementias and Schizophrenia

Characteristic patterns of abnormality are seen in the dementias and schizophrenia when patients are imaged with Tc-99m-HMPAO. Patients with **Alzheimer's disease** have reductions in regional cerebral blood flow in the temporal, parietal, and occasionally frontal regions. The sensitivity and specificity of this approach in diagnosing Alzheimer's disease are about 83% and

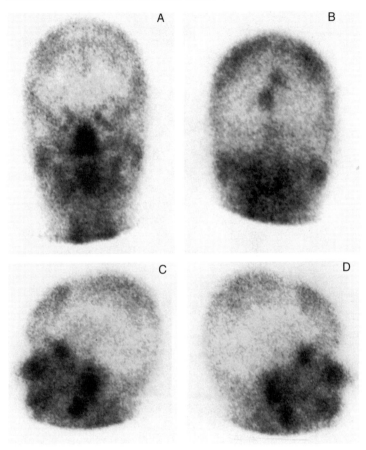

Figure 8-5. *continued*

60%, respectively. In patients with **multi-infarct dementia** the defects are randomly distributed. Severe reduction in frontal lobe perfusion is characteristic of **Pick's disease.**

Dementia has been detected from 65 to 87% of **AIDS** patients. Although AIDS patients may develop opportunistic infections of the brain, the dementia appears to be caused in almost all cases by the HIV infection. The associated findings seen with SPECT imaging with I-123-IMP or Tc-99m-HMPAO are single or multiple cortical cerebral defects.

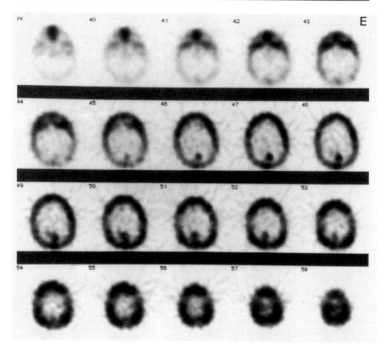

Figure 8-5. *continued*

Cocaine abuse is often associated with dementia, possibly on the basis of the vasoconstriction effects of the drug. In one study of 18 cocaine drug users, all had mild or moderate dementia, and 16 had abnormal Tc-99m-HMPAO studies characterized by small focal defects in the infraperitoneal, temporal, anterofrontal cortex, and basal ganglia.

The use of Tc-99m-HMPAO in the evaluation of **schizophrenia** is controversial. Two patterns of abnormality have been described. In the first, there is increased uptake in the caudate nuclei sometimes associated with increased uptake in the temporal lobes. In the second pattern, decreased uptake is seen in the frontal lobes. However, in a comparison of schizophrenic patients with normal subjects, neither of these findings was confirmed, but rather somewhat decreased uptake in the left temporal cortex was found in schizophrenic patients. Whether the

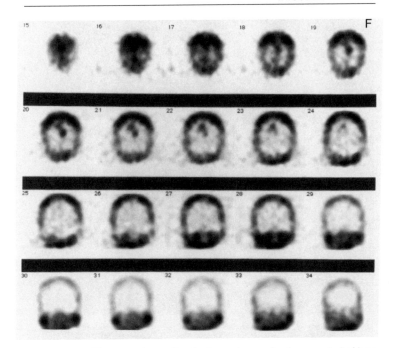

Figure 8-5. Tl-201 study positive for tumor in a patient suspected of having either lymphoma or infection. Planar views (**A,** ant.; **B,** post.; **C,** left lat.; **D,** right lat.) reveal a region of increased uptake in the posterior view only. SPECT axial (**E**) and coronal (**F**) views localize the uptake more precisely to both occipital lobes near the midline.

scintigraphic abnormalities reflect a primary brain abnormality or the effect of therapy is unknown.

Infection

Tc-99m-DTPA scintigraphy is very sensitive for focal infection. **Abscesses** are currently more frequently evaluated with computed tomography because it provides additional anatomic information. However, in cases where computed tomography is equivocal, In-111-granulocyte scintigraphy is useful to distinguish abscess from noninfectious focal lesions. Following the injection of In-111granulocytes, imaging is carried out at 4 and 24 hours.

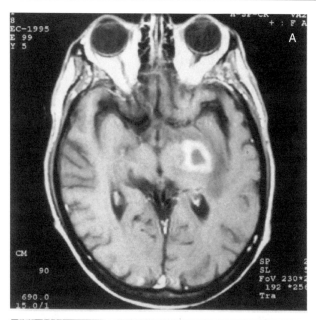

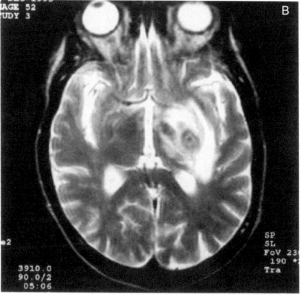

Figure 8-6. *continued*

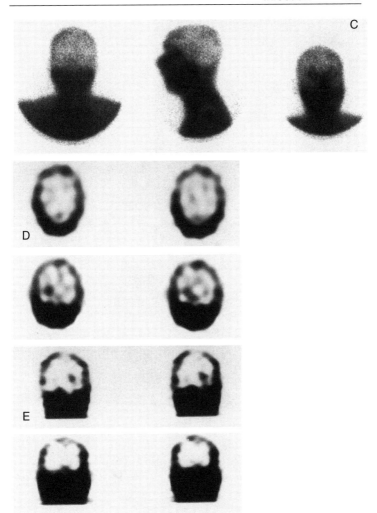

Figure 8-6. Tl-201 study positive for tumor in a patient suspected of having either lymphoma or infection. T1-weighted **(A)** and T2-weighted **(B)** MRI images show an abnormal focus in the left thalamus. This lesion is not clearly seen on posterior, left lateral, or anterior planar views **(C)**. SPECT axial **(D)** and coronal **(E)** views show increased uptake in the left thalamus.

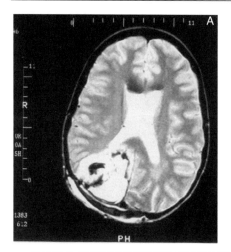

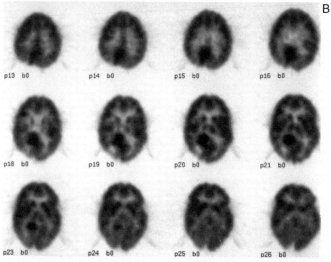

Figure 8-7. High-grade astrocytoma. **(A)** Following surgery and chemotherapy, an MRI reveals residual occipital abnormal tissue. **(B)** Axial slices from an F-18-FDG PET study show intense uptake in the abnormality detected on MRI. This high level of metabolic activity suggests tumor rather than posttherapeutic changes. (Courtesy of Donald Schauwecker, M.D., Indianapolis.)

The early diagnosis of **herpes** and **syphilis** brain infections is important because of the necessity of early therapy. Tc-99m-DTPA scintigraphy classically shows increased temporal uptake, sometimes with involvement of the parietal or frontal lobes (Fig. 8-8). The sensitivity of planar scintigraphy is 92% and may be higher when SPECT imaging is used with Tc-99m-DTPA. The sensitivity of CT scanning for herpes and syphilitis is 79%.

Trauma

Computed tomography has become the mainstay of imaging evaluation of the brain in head trauma. Tc-99m-DTPA scintigraphy remains useful in the evaluation of **chronic subdural hematoma.** The sensitivity for this condition is greater than 90%. The findings consist of crescentic increased uptake near the hematoma on delayed images and occasionally a peripheral mass effect on the perfusion portion of the study (Fig. 8-9).

Tc-99m-HMPAO SPECT imaging in **acute trauma** shows decreased uptake in injured brain. The sensitivity is greater than that of computed tomography, and the lesions seen on SPECT appear larger than the same lesions seen on CT. Abnormal brain

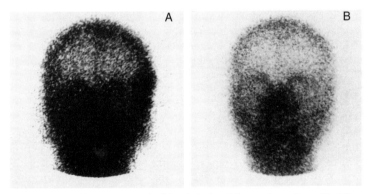

Figure 8-8. Herpes encephalitis. Anterior 2-hour views from Tc-99m-DTPA studies. This immunocompromised patient developed signs of left temporal lobe encephalopathy. **(A)** The initial study shows increased tracer uptake in the region of the left temporal lobe. This abnormality was determined to be herpes encephalitis. **(B)** A follow-up study several weeks later is normal.

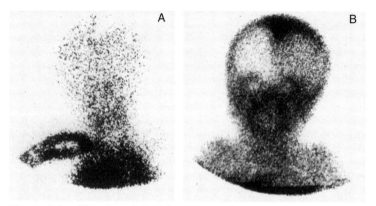

Figure 8-9. Chronic subdural hematoma. Selected anterior perfusion image **(A)** and 2-hour delayed image **(B)** from a Tc-99m-DTPA study. The perfusion image shows a photon- deficient region compressing the brain near the vertex, primarily on the left. The delayed image shows intensely increased uptake near the subdural hematoma adjacent to the vertex, and diffusely minimally increased uptake in the left cerebral hemisphere, possibly the result of contusion.

is characterized by focally increased or decreased uptake or diffusely decreased uptake (right to left hemispheric asymmetry or reversal of the normal, slightly higher uptake in the frontal lobes relative to the occipital lobes). Prognosis is poor when lesions are large, multiple, or located in the brain stem.

Epilepsy

Intractable **temporal lobe seizures** can be treated with surgical ablation of the seizure focus. The potential value of SPECT imaging is the localization of the seizure focus. Reports have varied, but there is general agreement that the seizure focus corresponds to a region of decreased perfusion on Tc-99m-HMPAO imaging. The sensitivity of SPECT imaging in the setting of epilepsy appears to be about 15%, although SPECT has been reported to be useful in localizing the seizure focus in about 70% of patients eventually having surgery. These figures are based on interictal imaging, and sensitivities for the much less convenient interictal approach may be significantly higher. These figures apply to adults, and the use of SPECT in children is less well defined.

Cerebral Palsy

SPECT brain imaging has been proposed as a method to evaluate the brains in children with cerebral palsy. The reasoning is that imaging could be used for prognostication and to direct early therapy. Tc-99m-HMPAO has shown hypoperfusion in regions corresponding to clinically detectable focal defects with greater sensitivity than CT. Because low doses are necessary in children, image quality is reduced; quantitative analysis of the images is necessary.

Cerebral Spinal Fluid Shunts, Leaks, And Obstructions

Shunts to relieve hydrocephalus drain cerebrospinal fluid (CSF) from the lateral ventricles into the right atrium or peritoneal cavity. The patency of the shunt and its associated reservoir and valve can be assessed with scintigraphy. One hundred uCi of a Tc-99m-labeled pharmaceutical such as DTPA or pertechnetate is injected into the reservoir. Subsequent continuous digital imaging of the reservoir yields a time–activity function that can be used to calculate CSF shunt flow in milliliters per minute. This calculation depends on knowledge of parameters of the shunt system that affect flow and that vary considerably among shunt systems. Normal CSF production in the adult is 0.4 to 0.5 mL/min, and a lower limit of normal for flow through a shunt has been suggested as 0.1 mL/min. Obtaining a precise numerical value for shunt flow is difficult, but several nonquantitative guidelines are available. First, the time–activity function of the reservoir should approximate a monoexponential function. Intermittent flow suggests shunt malfunction. Patients should be studied recumbent after having remained recumbent for 45 minutes to 2 hours before the onset of the study. Following the recumbent study a repeat study in the upright position can be performed; the resulting time–activity function should have a significantly shorter halftime than the recumbent one. Radioactivity in the abdomen, usually seen within 1 hour with normally functioning shunts, should disperse rather than remain confined near the catheter tip. Confinement suggests partial obstruction around the catheter tip.

CSF leaks may result from trauma or surgery and can be imaged following the injection of 0.5 mCi (18.5 Mbq) of In-111-DTPA

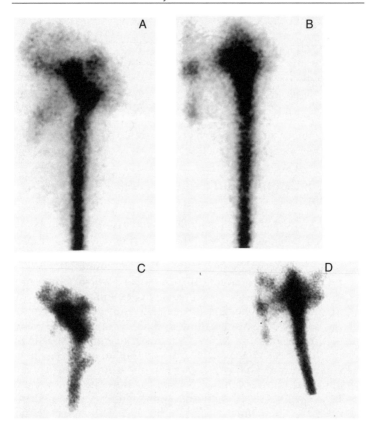

Figure 8-10. CFS leak; basilar skull fracture. All images were obtained 6 hours following intrathecal injection of In-111-DTPA. Right lateral **(A)** and anterior **(B)** views over the skull and neck were done to evaluate right-sided otorrhea shortly after a basilar skull fracture was sustained in an automobile accident. The radioactivity on the right side of the patient's face is CSF leaking into a wet dressing. A repeat study **(C, D)** shows residual leakage following a surgical attempt to repair the leak.

into the lumbar intrathecal space (Figs. 8-10, 8-11). In the case of basilar skull fracture, a suspected leak can be evaluated with a combination of scintigraphic imaging and the measurement of radioactivity in absorptive pledgets placed in the nose at the time of injection of tracer into the intrathecal space. Following the injection of In-111-DTPA into the lumbar intrathecal space, images of the head are obtained every hour until clear visualization of the

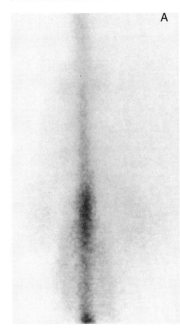
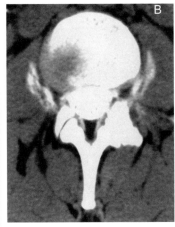

Figure 8-11. CFS leak following surgery. **(A)** Posterior view 2 hours after lumbar intrathecal injection of In-111-DTPA shows extravasation of tracer bilaterally parallel to the spine. **(B)** A selected image from a CT myelogram shows extravasated contrast medium between tissue planes.

basilar cisterns is obtained. After an additional 1 to 3 hours, images are obtained to search for a leak, and the pledgets are removed. Pledget radioactivity is measured and expressed in counts per minute per gram weight of the fluid absorbed by the pledgets. Pledget radioactivity greater than 1.3 times that of serum drawn at the time of pledget removal is suggestive of a CSF leak.

Obstructive communicating normal pressure hydrocephalus is a syndrome of gait disturbance, dementia, and incontinence associated with normal pressure hydrocephalus. The foramina of Monroe and Magendie are patent, but CSF flow is blocked by peripheral obstruction, usually at the level of the temporal or parietal lobes. The obstruction is frequently the result of scarred hematomas or meningitis, although meningeal tumor can also obstruct CSF flow. This condition can be distinguished from the normal pressure hydrocephalus of simple **atrophy** with CSF scintigraphy (Table 8-1). One-half millicurie of In-111-DTPA is injected into the lumbar intrathecal space. Images are performed at 2, 6, and 24 hours. In the normal patient, radioactivity reaches

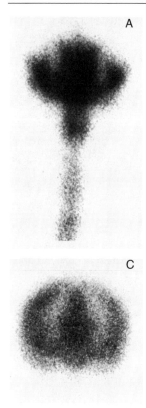

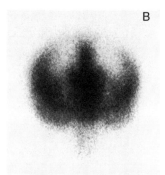

Figure 8-12. Cerebral atrophy. Anterior views from an In-111-DTPA cysternogram at 6 hours **(A)**, 24 hours **(B)**, and 48 hours **(C)** show intense radioactivity in dilated lateral ventricles and delayed progression of the tracer front to the vertex. These findings are the result of increased CSF space volume without obstruction.

the vertex by 24 hours and is not seen to a significant degree in the lateral ventricles. In simple atrophy, radioactivity reaches the vertex at greater than 24 hours, and radioactivity may be seen in the lateral ventricles (Fig. 8-12). In obstructive normal-pressure com-

Table 8-1. Comparison of Scintigraphic Findings in Atrophy, Obstructive Communicating Normal-Pressure Hydrodephalus (NPH), and Normal. Transit time is time of arrival of the visible radioactive front at vertex.

	Ventricles	Transit Time
Atrophy	Dilated	>_48 hr
NPH	Dilated	(peripheral block)
	≥ 48 hr (block near arachuoidal granulations)
Normal	Not visualized	24 hr

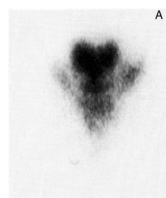

A

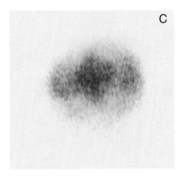

Figure 8-13. Obstructive communicating normal-pressure hydrocephalus. Anterior views from an In-111-DTPA cysternogram at 4 hours **(A),** 24 hours **(B),** and 48 hours **(C)** show intense radioactivity in dilated lateral ventricles and failure of the visible tracer front to progress beyond bilateral partial obstructions at the parietal level. This patient was a professional boxer with gait abnormality, dementia, and urinary incontinence. The cause of the obstruction was very likely scarring of the subarachnoid space secondary to multiple small bleeds.

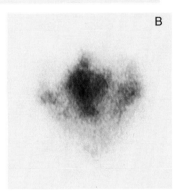

B

C

municating hydrocephalus, the leading edge of radioactivity that ascends around the cerebral hemispheres, changes caliber and intensity abruptly at the point of obstruction, and minimal, if any radioactivity is seen beyond the obstruction even on images delayed more than 24 hours (Fig. 8-13). Reflux of radioactivity into the lateral ventricles is frequent.

CSF flow can be disrupted by **meningeal tumor.** Scintigraphy can be used to characterize the flow dynamics to aid in decisions about shunts and intrathecal chemotherapy (Fig. 8–14).

Eyes

Scintigraphic techniques have been investigated for the evaluation of diabetic retinopathy and ocular tumors. These approaches have not been widely accepted. However, radionu-

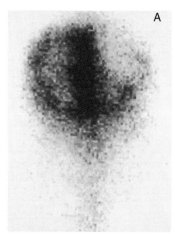

A

Figure 8-14. Metastatic breast cancer to meninges. **(A)** Anterior view from an In-111-DTPA cysternogram 24 hours after injection shows reduced CSF flow over the left cerebral hemisphere. **(B)** Enhancing tumor is confirmed on a CT image. Intrathecal chemotherapy was contemplated in this patient, but the scintigraphy suggested that the therapeutic agent would not reach the tumor.

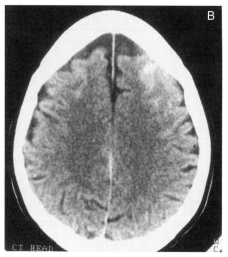

B

clide dacryoscintigraphy is occasionally used to evaluate for obstruction of the lacrimal duct. From 50 to 100 uCi of Tc-99m-pertechnetate in 10 μL of normal saline are instilled into the conjunctional sac. Image acquisition with a gamma camera fitted with a pinhole collimator is done every 10 to 20 seconds for 2 minutes and then at 5, 10, 15, and 20 min. Tracer normally moves medially through the lacrimal canaliculi to the

Figure 8-15. Normal dacryoscintigram. **(A)** Anterior image done 5 minutes after administration of Tc-99m-pertechnetate into the conjunctival sacs visualizes both nasolacrimal apparatuses. **(B)** The diagram identifies the conjunctival sac (CS), canaliculi (C), nasolacrimal bulb (B), and naso-lacrimal duct (D).

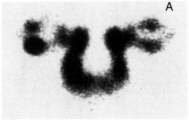
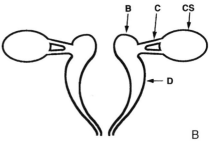

lacrimal sac, which is visualized within seconds of instillation. The lacrimal duct is visualized within a few minutes (Fig. 8-15). Obstruction, if complete, prevents these structures from being visualized. Partial obstruction causes a delay of visualization on the involved side (Figs. 8-16, 8-17). Symmetry is an important criterion in the evaluation for obstruction, and test sensitivity is reduced in partial symmetrical obstruction.

Figure 8-16. Unilateral naso-lacrimal lacrimal duct obstruction. At 15 minutes this anterior dacryoscintigram shows a normal left and obstructed right nasal lacrimal duct.

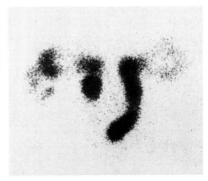

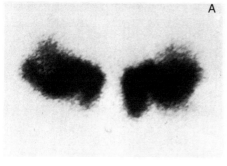

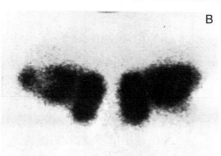

Figure 8-17. Bilateral nasal lacrimal duct obstruction. Anterior dacryoscintigraphic images at 5 minutes **(A)** and 15 minutes **(B)** fail to show the distal portions of the nasolacrimal ducts.

References

Abdel-Dayem HM, Sadek SA, Kouris K, et al.: Changes in cerebral perfusion after acute head injury: comparison of CT with Tc-99m HM-PAO SPECT. *Radiology* 1987;165:221-226.

Ackerman ES, Tumeh SS, Charron M, English R and Deresiewicv R: Viral encephalitis: imaging with SPECT. *Clinical Nuclear Medicine* 1988;13:640-643.

Biersack HJ, Grunwald F, Kropp J: Single photon emission computed tomography imaging of brain tumors. *Semin Nucl Med* 1991;21(1):2-10.

Bonte FJ, Hom J, Tintner R, Weiner MF: Single photon tomography in Alzheimer's disease and the dementias. *Semin Nucl Med* 1990;20(4):342-352.

Brendel AJ, Wynchank S, Castel JP, Barat JL, Leccia F, Ducassou D: Cerebrospinal shunt flow in adults: radionuclide quantitation with emphasis on patient position. *Radiology* 1983;149:815-818.

Cohen MB, Lake RR, Graham S, et al.: Quantitative iodine-123 IMP imaging of brain perfusion in schizophrenia. *J Nucl Med* 1989;30:1616-1620.

Cowan RJ: Conventional radionuclide brain imaging in the era of transmission and emission tomography. *Semin Nucl Med* 1986;16(1):63-73.

Denays R, Tondeur M, Toppet V, et al.: Cerebral palsy: initial experience with Tc-99m HMPAO SPECT of the brain. *Radiology* 1990;175:111-116.

Denffer HV, Pabst HW: Lacrimal dacryoscintigraphy. *Semin Nucl Med* 1984;14(1):8-15.

Devous MD, Leroy RF, Homan RW: Single photon emission computed tomography in epilepsy. *Semin Nucl Med* 1990;20(4):325-341.

Holman BL, Carvalho PA, Mendelson J, et al.: Brain perfusion is abnormal in cocaine-dependent polydrug users: a study using technetium-99m-HMPAO and ASPECT. *J Nucl Med* 1991;32:1206-1210.

Kramer EL, Sanger JJ: Brain imaging in acquired immunodeficiency syndrome dementia complex. *Semin Nucl Med* 1990;20(4):353-363.

Kuni CC, Rogge DM: Radionuclide brain perfusion studies in suspected brain death. *Clin Nucl Med* 1986;11(8):551-555.

Laurin NR, Driedger AA, Hurwitz GA, et al.: Cerebral perfusion imaging with technetium-99m HM-PAO in brain death and severe central nervous system injury. *J Nucl Med* 1989;30:1627-1635.

Lee VW, Hauck RM, Morrison MC, Peng TT, Fischer E, Carter A: Scintigraphy evaluation of brain death: significance of sagittal sinus visualization. *J Nucl Med* 1987;28:1279-1283.

Maurer AH, Siegel JA, Comerota AJ, Morgan WA, Johnson MH: SPECT quantification of cerebral ischemia before and after carotid endarterectomy. *J Nucl Med* 1990;31(8):1412-1420.

McKusick KA, Malmud LS, Kordela PA, Wagner HN Jr: Radionuclide cisternography: normal values for nasal secretion of intrathecally injected 111-In-DTPA. *J Nucl Med* 1973;14(12):933-934.

Rowe CC, Berkovic SF, Austin MC, et al.: Visual and quantitative analysis of interictal SPECT with technetium-99m-HMPAO in temporal lobe epilepsy. *J Nucl Med* 1991;32:1688-1694.

Ruiz A, Ganz WI, Post JD: Use of thallium-201 brain SPECT to differentiate cerebral lymphoma from toxoplasma encephalitis in AIDS patients. *Am J Neuroradiol* 1994;15:1885-1894.

Schmidt KG, Rasmussen JW, Frederiksen PB, Kock-Jensen C, Pedersen NT: Indium-111-granulocyte scintigraphy in brain abscess diagnosis: limitations and pitfalls. *J Nucl Med* 1990;31:1121-1127.

Teaching editorial. Radionuclide tests of cerebral fluid shunt patency. *J Nucl Med* 1984;25(1):112-114.

Van Heertum RL, O'Connell RA: Functional brain imaging in the evaluation of psychiatric illness. *Semin Nucl Med* 1991;21(1):24-39.

Chapter 9

Lungs

Pulmonary Embolism

Clinical Features

Pulmonary thromboembolism (PE) is a common and lethal condition. Autopsy data suggest that the incidence of PE in the United States is about 630,000 cases per year. Eleven percent of these victims die within 1 hour. Of those who survive longer than 1 hour, diagnosis is made and appropriate therapy is instituted in 29%, and of these patients 92% survive. Of the undiagnosed victims, 70% survive.

Sixty-four percent of patients at autopsy have evidence of remote or recent PE manifested by minute foci of organized thrombus to massive acute thromboembolism. Autopsy series in the past demonstrated that PE played a major role in from 9 to 21% of deaths. The rate of PE as the cause of death has decreased as anticoagulation therapy has increased and is now probably between 3 and 4% of autopsied patients. Thirty-one percent of patients with PE are found to have pulmonary infarction at autopsy; this fraction is probably much smaller in survivors. Infarction appears to be more likely when pulmonary artery branches with diameters of 3 mm or less are occluded than when larger arteries are occluded. These observations, along with the relatively inaccurate signs and symptoms in PE, make an accurate test desirable.

Physiology

PE usually does not cause infarction, because the bronchial arteries provide the lung with a second blood supply. PE without infarction initially reduces pulmonary arterial blood flow to the involved region to essentially zero. Recanalization may result in significant return of pulmonary perfusion as soon as 24 hours after the embolic event. PE, even without infarction, may result

Table 9–1. Pathophysiology of PE

	V	P	CXR
PE	N	O	Clear
INFARCT	O	O	Density
PNEUMONIA	O	O	Density
COPD	↓	↓	Clear

The minimal reflexive decrease in ventilation that occurs in PE without infarction is usually not an important factor in the interpretation of lung scans and is ignored here. V = ventilation, P = perfusion, N = normal, O = absent. ↓ = decreased, CXR = chest x-ray.

in a small degree of reflex decrease in ventilation in the involved region. When PE causes infarction, ventilation in the infarcted lung diminishes significantly because of the presence of fluid and cells in the involved alveoli and bronchi.

Nonthromboembolic lung diseases such as pneumonia and chronic obstructive disease (COPD) in which ventilation is decreased cause decreased pulmonary arterial perfusion through the hypoxic vasoconstriction response. This response is strong, and regional lung diseases—including those not associated with chest film densities—cause significant regional decreases in pulmonary arterial perfusion as measured scintigraphically. These concepts are summarized in Table 9–1.

Notice that a test that measures regional ventilation and regional pulmonary perfusion in conjunction with the chest x-ray can diagnose pulmonary embolism without infarction as a distinct entity. The same test cannot distinguish pulmonary embolism with infarction from pneumonia. COPD, however, can be distinguished from the other three conditions.

Technique

Perfusion imaging is accomplished by the intravenous injection of several hundred thousand particles of macroaggregated albumin or albumin microspheres labeled with 5 mCi of Tc-99m. Injection is done with the patient recumbent to minimize the effects of gravity on regional pulmonary perfusion. Imaging is done in the anterior, posterior, both lateral, and all four oblique projections. The patient may be upright or recumbent for perfusion imaging, but the same position should be used for the ventilation imaging.

Ventilation imaging is performed with either a radioactive gas, usually Xe-133, or a labeled aerosol, usually Tc-99m-DTPA. The 80-keV predominant energy peak of Xe-133 necessitates that ventilation imaging is done before perfusion imaging. Twenty to 30 mCi of Xe-133 are injected into a closed airway immediately before the patient takes in a single deep breath and holds it. During this period of breath-holding an image is acquired. This initial image is compared with the perfusion images. Following the single-breath image, the patient breathes quietly with a closed system containing a mixture of Xe-133 and air. A video display of the image being acquired during equilibrium is monitored. When wash-in of slowly ventilating regions reaches equilibrium, a 500,000-count image is obtained. Then, at 30- to 60-second intervals, washout images are obtained using the same acquisition time as for the equilibrium images. In most cases all the ventilation images are obtained in the posterior projection. Regions that ventilate slowly will show decreased intensity on the initial single-breath image, will fill in with equilibrium, and will wash out slowly. The washout image therefore can be compared with the perfusion images when the patient is incapable of breath-holding for the initial image. In this case, scintigraphically hot regions are assumed to represent regions that would have been cold in a successful single-breath image.

The 5.3-day half-life of Xe-133 is convenient, but the 80-keV energy is somewhat low for ideal imaging. Xe-127 offers the advantage of higher-energy photons (172, 203, and 375 keV), allowing for postperfusion ventilation imaging. However, these energies are higher than ideal for high-quality imaging. The half-life of Xe-127 is 36 days, longer than ideal. Kr-81m has a photon energy of 190 keV and a half-life of 13 days, making this a nearly ideal gas for ventilation imaging. Xe-127 and Kr-81m are both expensive and uncommonly used for this reason.

In recent years several manufacturers have perfected single-use Tc-99m-DTPA-aerosol generators. The patient inhales the aerosol for several minutes and is monitored with a calibrated gamma camera to determine when the inhalation should be stopped for a desired dose level. Because the labels of the aerosol and the MAA used for perfusion are both Tc-99m, a dosage difference factor of 2 to 5 is used to prevent the first study from interfering significantly with the second. Either order can be used, and this decision depends somewhat on the local patient population. When the likelihood of pulmonary embolism and other pulmonary disease is low, perfusion imaging can be done first. If perfusion is normal, ventilation imaging need not be done. The advantage of preperfusion ventilation imaging is that the perfusion image is then the one done with the higher dose of tracer and therefore the one that results in images of higher quality. The major advantage of aerosol imaging is that once the aerosol has been inhaled, its distribution does not change significantly for as long as an hour. This stability allows for imaging in all the same projections as are used in perfusion imaging. A disadvantage of aerosol imaging is that central airway deposition of aerosol occurs in chronic lung diseases and may detract from image quality.

Interpretation

The concepts in Table 9–1 can be used as a first step in understanding the interpretation of scintigraphic ventilation/perfusion studies. Theoretically, the probability of pulmonary embolism is high in a region that is normal in ventilation images and shows absent radioactivity in perfusion images. The likelihood of PE in a region of lung should be low when the region shows normal perfusion on perfusion images. A region of lung that has a radiographic density, no ventilation, and no perfusion is indeterminate in likelihood for PE because the cause of the abnormality may be infarction or nonthromboembolic focal disease such as pneumonia. Several large studies have addressed the questions of the sizes and severities of regional abnormalities that suggest different probabilities of PE. Table 9–2 summarizes the criteria as recommended by McNeil, Biello, Klingensmith, and the Prospective Investigation of Pulmonary Embolism Detection (PIOPED) group. There are only minimal differences in the accuracies of these techniques. Figures 9–1 through 9–12 illustrate these principles.

In transplanted lungs and in the lungs of patients with COPD or pulmonary hypertension, the hypoxic vasoconstriction response is frequently blunted or absent. In these lungs, a ventilatory abnormality may not lead to the perfusion abnormalities encountered in native lungs; in the resulting reverse mismatch,

text continued on page 199

Table 9–2.

Category	McNeal	Biello	PIOPED	Klingensmith
Normal	Normal P	Normal P	Normal P	Normal P; CXR clear
Low probability	• One segmental or subsegmental V-P mismatch, CXR clear • V-P matches alone • Multiple subsegmental V-P mismatches, CXR clear	• Small V-P mismatches • V-P matches without corresponding desities on CXR • Perfusion defect substantially smaller then CXR density • Severe COPD • Single medium V-P mismatch	• Small P defects (any number) and normal CXR • Matched V-P defects with clear CXR • P defect with larger CXR abnormality	• <10% certainty of V-P mismatch
Intermediate	• Mixed V-P match and mismatch		• Abnormality not classifiable to other categories • Single matched V-P defect with clear CXR • V-P mismatched defects in .5–2 segments total	• 10% to 90 % certainty of V-P mismatch
Indeterminate	• Perfusion defect with matched density on CXR	• Perfusion defect with matched density on CXR		
High	• Single lobar or larger V-P mismatch with normal CXR • Multiple segmental or larger V-P mismatches with normal CXR	• Single large V-P mismatch • Perfusion defect larger than density on CXR • Multiple medium or large V-P mismatches without matched density on CXR	• V-P mismatched defects in ≥ 2 segments total	• CXR density with infarct; <90% certainty of V-P mismatch • >90% certainty of V-P mismatch

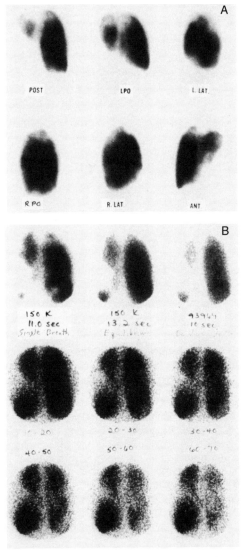

Figure 9-1. *continued*

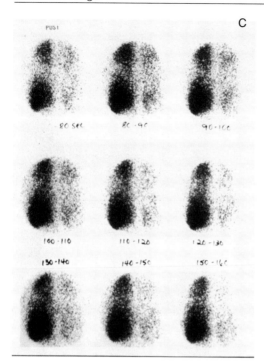

Figure 9–1. Chronic obstructive disease. **(A)** Perfusion images show essentially absent perfusion of the left lower lung. The remainder of the study shows inhomogeneous perfusion that is focally worse at the right apex. **(B)** and **(C)** The single-breath image (upper left) matches the perfusion study reasonably well. Washout images show focally delayed washout at the left apex and left lower lung. Regions that wash in slowly tend to wash out slowly. (The intensity level was increased, starting with the 10- to 20-second image.) Because of the widespread severe non-thromboembolic pulmonary disease and because of a small perfusion–ventilation mismatch at the left apex, this study was interpreted as indicating a moderate probability of PE.

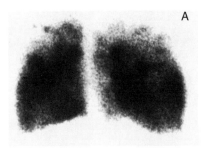

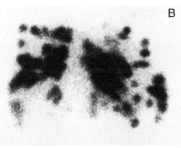

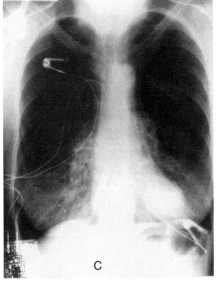

Figure 9–2. Chronic obstructive disease. **(A)** Posterior perfusion view shows diffusely inhomogeneous deposition of MAA, worst at the apices. **(B)** Posterior view of aerosol ventilation study shows diffuse, severely inhomogeneous deposition of aerosol. **(C)** The chest film is clear. Although a perfusion–ventilation mismatch is not apparent, the severe diffuse nonthromboembolic pulmonary abnormality makes moderate probability for PE the appropriate interpretation. Ventilation is diffusely worse than perfusion; such reverse mismatch is frequently seen in patients with COPD.

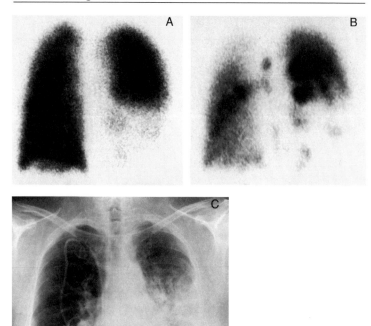

Figure 9–3. **(A)** Anterior perfusion and **(B)** aerosol ventilation views show a large matched left lower lung defect. **(C)** Whether a corresponding density on the chest x-ray represents infarction or nonthromboembolic disease such as pneumonia is indeterminate from this study. The appropriate interpretation for such a triple match is therefore indeterminate probability for PE.

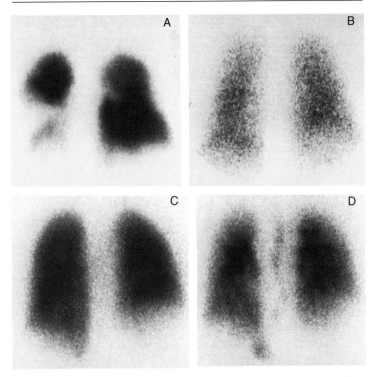

Figure 9–4. Resolving PE. **(A)** Several left lower lung segments show decreased perfusion in the posterior view. **(B)** Posterior single-breath Xenon ventilation shows normal ventilation in this region. Interpretation: high probability for PE. The patient underwent thrombolytic therapy. A repeat study 3 days later (posterior perfusion **(C)** and posterior aerosol ventilation **(D)**) shows resolution of the perfusion defects.

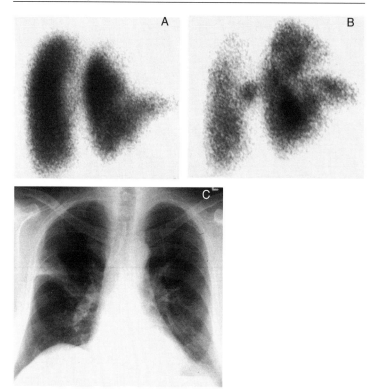

Figure 9–5. High probability for PE. **(A)** Right posterior oblique perfusion and **(B)** aerosol ventilation show right and left upper lobe perfusion–ventilation mismatches. **(C)** A density on the chest x-ray corresponds to decreased perfusion and ventilation in the anterior segment of the upper lobe; this segment is probably infarcted. The lateral segment of the middle lobe shows a perfusion–ventilation match with no chest film density; embolism in this segment is unlikely. **(D)** Doppler ultrasound examination of the left popliteal vein shows an echo-dense thrombus dilating the vein. Forward flow in this region is significantly diminished, and there is super-imposed artifact caused by pulsation of the adjacent artery.

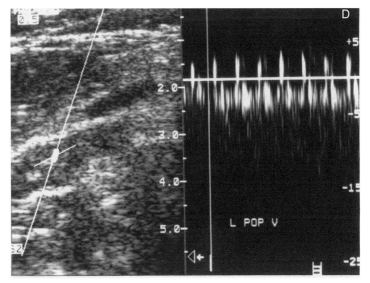

Figure 9-5. *continued*

scintigraphy shows relatively preserved perfusion in regions of decreased ventilation (Figs. 9–2, 9–7, and 9–12).

The sensitivity and specificity of ventilation–perfusion scintigraphy depend on the definitions of positive and negative test results. This issue was addressed in the PIOPED study. If a positive test is defined as any result other than normal (high, intermediate, or low probability), then the sensitivity is 98% and the specificity is 10%. If high- or intermediate-probability interpretations are considered a positive test result, then the sensitivity and specificity are 82 and 52%, respectively. If only a high-probability interpretation is accepted as a positive test result, then the sensitivity and specificity are 41 and 97%, respectively.

Roughly one-third of patients undergoing ventilation–perfusion scintigraphy will have a low-probability interpretation, another third will be indeterminate or intermediate, and the remaining third will be about evenly divided between normal or near-normal and high probability. Of patients with high-probability interpretations, 88% have been found by angiography to have PE. This figure drops to 33% for intermediate probability, 16% for low probability, and 9% for normal or near-normal interpretations. *text continued on page 203*

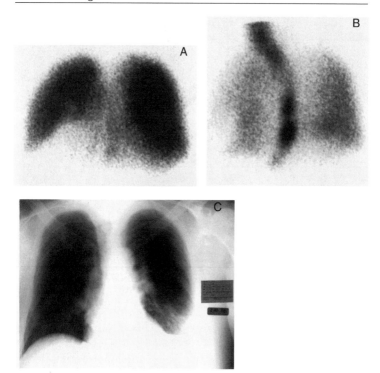

Figure 9–6. PE with infarction. **(A)** Posterior perfusion and **(B)** aerosol ventilation show a large perfusion defect involving the left posterior basilar and lateral basilar segments. A significantly smaller ventilation defect involves only the lateral basilar segment, and ventilation in the posterior basilar segment is preserved. **(C)** A density in the chest x-ray corresponds to the lateral basilar portion of the abnormality and probably represents an infarction.

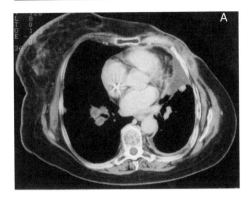

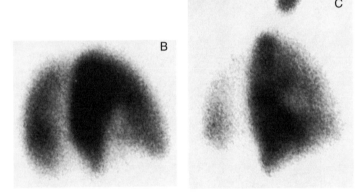

Figure 9–7. High probability for PE. **(A)** A contrast-enhanced computed tomographic examination was done to evaluate posttherapeutic changes in the left hemithorax in this patient with breast cancer and previous mastectomy and radiation therapy. Filling defects in large pulmonary arteries near the right hilum are surrounded by higher-density blood. This finding suggested pulmonary embolism, although the patient had no symptoms referable to the right hemithorax. RPO perfusion **(B)** and aerosol ventilation **(C)** show mismatched perfusion defects in the right anterior basilar segment and right posterior basilar segment. Reverse mismatches in the middle lobe and right upper lobe may reflect COPD.

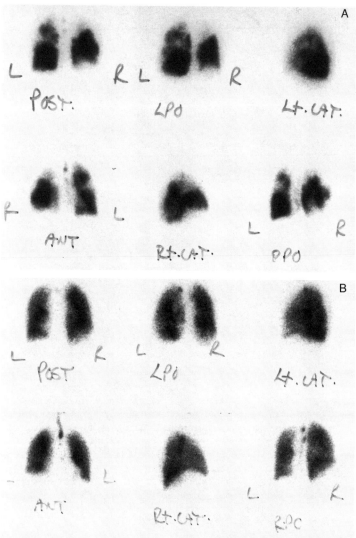

Figure 9-8. *continued*

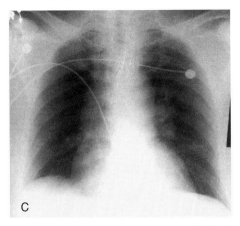

Figure 9–8. High probability for PE. **(A)** Perfusion and **(B)** aerosol ventilation show multiple segments of absent or significantly decreased perfusion with relatively intact ventilation. **(C)** The chest x-ray is clear.

Anticoagulation can reasonably be withheld from patients with normal scintigraphy and can be administered to patients with high-probability scintigraphy. Patients with intermediate- and sometimes low-probability interpretations may need additional studies such as lower-extremity venous Doppler ultrasound or pulmonary angiography. Angiography may be unnecessary when venous Doppler ultrasound shows lower-extremity deep venous thrombi.

Pulmonary arterial abnormalities other than PE can cause significant perfusion–ventilation mismatches. Pulmonary arteries that are abnormal congenitally or as a result of surgery may be associated with regions of abnormal pulmonary perfusion but intact ventilation (Figs. 9–13, 9–14). Tumor encasement of pulmonary arteries may lead to similar findings even in the absence of PE and should be suspected in cases of multiple congruent involved segments as the only perfusion defect. Vasculitis is usually diffuse but occasionally causes segmental perfusion–ventilation mismatches (Fig. 9–15). *text continued on page 208*

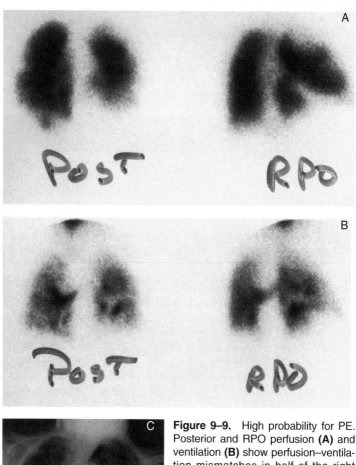

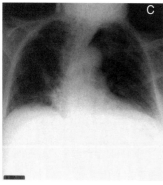

Figure 9–9. High probability for PE. Posterior and RPO perfusion **(A)** and ventilation **(B)** show perfusion–ventilation mismatches in half of the right anterior basilar segment, one-half of the lateral segment of the middle lobe, all of the right apical segment, and all of the left lateral basilar segment—for a total of the equivalent of three mismatched segments. **(C)** The chest x-ray shows patchy infiltrates in the right mid-lung and left base that do not affect the interpretation.

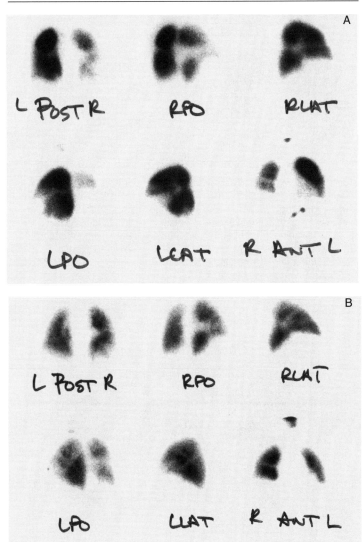

Figure 9-10. *continued*

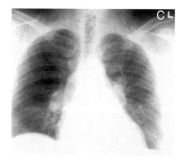

Figure 9–10. High probability for PE. **(A)** Perfusion and ventilation **(B)** images show several segmental mismatches. In addition, overall perfusion of the right lung relative to the left is significantly decreased, whereas overall ventilation is relatively symmetrical. These findings suggest a large, partially occluding thromboembolus in the right main pulmonary artery. **(C)** The chest film shows diffusely less parenchymal density in the right lung than the left along with a dilated proximal right pulmonary artery (Westermark's sign).

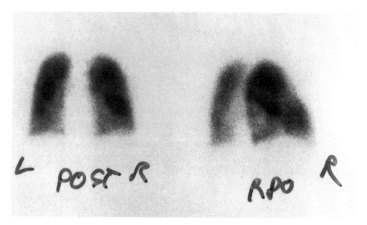

Figure 9–11. Stripe sign. A partial perfusion defect best seen in the RPO view involves the right posterior basilar and right lateral basilar segments. Although this defect might be suspect for pulmonary embolism, a peripheral margin of relatively preserved perfusion militates against embolism.

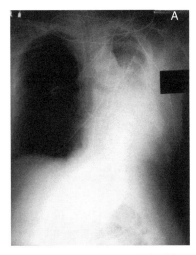

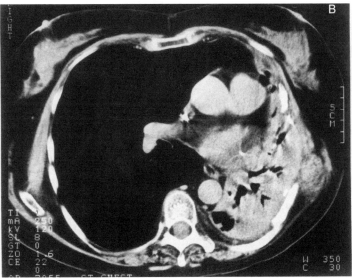

Figure 9-12. *continued*

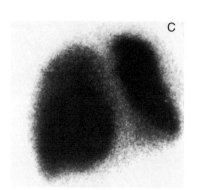

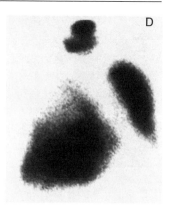

Figure 9–12. Transplanted lung, low probability for PE. This patient received a left lung transplant for severe COPD. **(A)** Chest film and **(B)** computed tomography show a density involving the lower left lung. The mediastinum is shifted to the left, and the left lung is compressed by the hyperinflated right lung. **(C)** Anterior aerosol image shows significantly decreased ventilation in the left lower lung. **(D)** Anterior perfusion image shows preserved perfusion in the left lower lung. The hypoxic vasoconstriction response is blunted or absent in transplanted lungs. This phenomenon is also frequently seen in COPD, as in this patient's right apex.

Fat and marrow emboli released from fractured large bones into the venous circulation may mimic thromboembolism clinically and scintigraphically. However, the more common pulmonary manifestation of embolic fat is local tissue damage caused by the breakdown of microscopic droplets of fat diffusely in the pulmonary microcirculation. The chest x-ray typically shows a diffuse interstitial infiltrate, and perfusion scintigraphy shows only minimal peripheral inhomogeneity or no abnormality (Fig. 9–16).

Airway Disease

Ventilation imaging with Tc-99m-DTPA aerosol or a radioactive gas such as Xe-133 can be used to assess regional ventilatory abnormalities in diseases that affect the bronchi, such as COPD (Figs. 9–1, 9–2) and cystic fibrosis (Fig. 9–17). Pulmonary

text continued on page 211

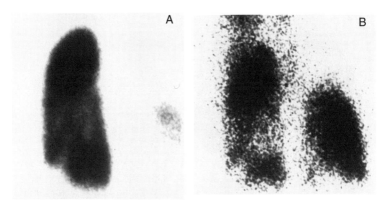

Figure 9–13. Postoperative tetralogy of Fallot; no PE. Pulmonary arterial flow to the right lung was surgically reduced. **(A)** Posterior perfusion and **(B)** ventilation images show the resulting perfusion–ventilation mismatch.

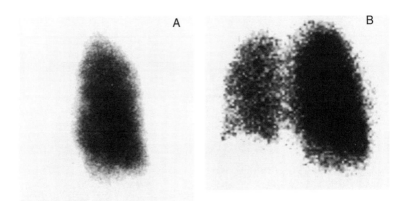

Figure 9–14. Agenesis of the left main pulmonary artery; no PE. **(A)** Posterior perfusion and **(B)** Xenon ventilation show absent pulmonary perfusion to the left lung but relatively intact ventilation. The involved left lung is congenitally smaller than the right, as is typical in this condition.

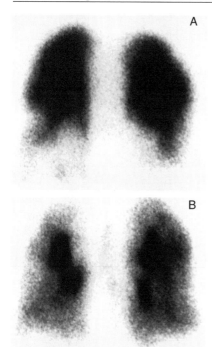

Figure 9–15. Rheumatoid arthritis; no PE. **(A)** Posterior perfusion and **(B)** aerosol ventilation images show multiple lower-lung large areas of mismatch. This patient proved to have rheumatoid lung disease without pulmonary embolism.

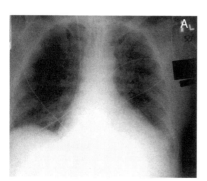
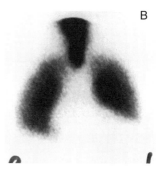

Figure 9–16. Fat emboli syndrome. This patient sustained large bone fractures in an automobile accident 2 days before the chest film. **(A)** There are diffuse bilateral interstitial infiltrates. **(B)** Anterior perfusion image from a study performed at the bedside is normal except for diffuse peripheral inhomogeneity. Radioactivity in the oropharynx resulted from a failed aerosol ventilation study.

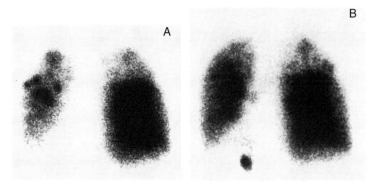

Figure 9–17. Cystic fibrosis; response to therapy. Posterior aerosol ventilation studies. **(A)** The initial study was done at the time of admission to the hospital during an exacerbation. Aerosol deposition in the left lung and right apex is markedly reduced and inhomogeneous. The focal intense deposits of aerosol in the left lung may represent regions of bronchiectasis. **(B)** Following 3 weeks of therapy, the left lung has improved significantly but the right apex has not.

function testing (PFT) yields a global measure of lung function, but therapeutic decisions may depend on knowledge of regional abnormalities. For example, a cystic fibrosis patient with overall improvement in treated bronchitis but with worsening in one region may have improved pulmonary function testing. The PFT alone could inappropriately lead to cessation of antibiotics.

Pulmonary Arteriovenous Shunts

If abnormal communications exist between the pulmonary arteries and pulmonary veins, Tc-99m-MAA injected into a systemic vein will not be extracted from the blood by the pulmonary capillary bed with 100% efficiency. The tracer that bypasses the lungs will enter the systemic arterial circulation, and images will show radioactivity in the brain, heart, kidneys, and to a lesser degree, other organs. Causes of shunting that can be evaluated with Tc-99m-MAA imaging include intracardiac shunts (Fig. 9–18), arteriovenous malformations, and hepatopulmonary syndrome (Fig. 9–19).

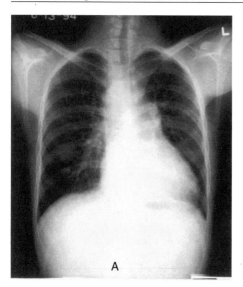

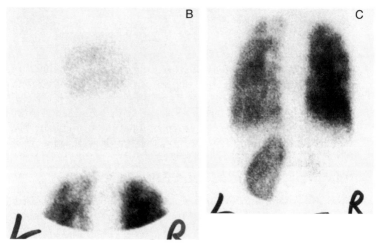

Figure 9–18. VSD Eisenmenger's syndrome with right-to-left shunt. Chest x-ray **(A)** shows cardiomegaly, enlarged proximal pulmonary arteries, and a right aortic arch. The patient was found to have a VSD. Posterior perfusion images over the head, neck, and upper thorax **(B)** and over the thorax and upper abdomen **(C)** show significant uptake of MAA in the brain and solitary left kidney in addition to the lungs.

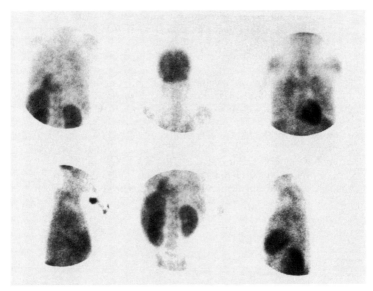

Figure 9–19. Hepatopulmonary syndrome. This patient had severe cirrhosis with secondary intrapulmonary pulmonary artery to pulmonary venous shunting. MAA perfusion images show some lung uptake, but significant intrapulmonary shunting is indicated by uptake in the brain, myocardium, enlarged spleen, and kidneys.

Suggested Readings

Biello DR: Radiological (scintigraphic) evaluation of patients with suspected pulmonary thromboembolism. *JAMA* 1987;257:3257.

Dismuke SE, Wagner EH: Pulmonary embolism as a cause of death. *JAMA* 1986;255:2039–2042.

Freiman DG, Suyemoto J, Wessler S: Frequency of pulmonary embolism in man. *N Engl J Med* 1965;272:1278–1280.

Gottschalk A, Juni JE, Sostman HD, et al: Ventilation-perfusion scintigraphically in the PIOPED study. Part I. Data collection and tabulation. *J Nucl Med* 1993;34:1109–1118.

Klingensmith WC, Holt SA: Lung scan interpretation: A physiologic, user-friendly approach. *J Nucl Med* 1992;33:1417–1422.

Krowka MJ: Hepatopulmonary syndrome: An evolving perspective in the era of liver transplantation. *Hepatology* 1990;11:138–142.

Kuni CC, Budd JR, Regelmann WE, du cret RP, Boudreau RJ: Comparison of Tc-99m DTPA aerosol ventilation studies with pulmonary function testing in cystic fibrosis. *Clin Nucl Med* 1993;18:15–18.

Kuni CC, du Cret RP, Nakhleh RE, Boudreau RJ: Reverse mismatch between perfusion and aerosol ventilation in transplanted lungs. *Clin Nucl Med* 1993;18:313–317.

The PIOPED Investigators: Value of the ventilation/perfusion scan in acute pulmonary embolism. Results of the prospective investigation of pulmonary embolism diagnosis (PIOPED). *JAMA* 1990;263:2753–2759.

Webber MM, Gomes AS, Roe D, La Fontaine RL, Hawkins RA: Comparison of Biello, McNeil, and PIOPED criteria for the diagnosis of pulmonary emboli on lung scans. *AJR* 1990;154:975–981.

Wellman HN: Pulmonary thromboembolism: current status report on the role of nuclear medicine. *Semin Nucl Med* 1986;16:236–274.

Chapter 10

Inflammation and Tumor Imaging

The first intended clinical application of gallium was as a bone-imaging agent. In the late 1960s it was applied to tumor imaging, then, in the early 1970s it became an agent for imaging of inflammation and infection. Ga-67 is produced by bombardment of Zn-68 in a cyclotron. The product is an isotope with a physical half-life of 78 hours and an electron capture decay scheme that produces four photopeaks at 93, 185, 300, and 394 keV. The 93-keV photopeak is the most abundant (40%), and the lowest three photopeaks are generally used for imaging. The properties of Ga-67 citrate after injection are similar to those of ferric ion. After Ga-67 dissociates there is binding of the radioisotope to lactoferrin, transferrin, and siderophores. Degranulation of neutrophils causes release of lactoferrin, which then results in binding of Ga-67. Increased vascular permeability increases delivery of Ga-67 to sites of inflammation and infection. Direct binding of Ga-67 to leukocytes and bacteria does occur but is not the dominant cause of accumulation of the radioisotope at sites of inflammation. Metabolism of lactoferrin and transferrin causes prominent accumulation of Ga-67 in the liver.

After a standard dose of 3 to 5 mCi is injected approximately 20% of the Ga-67 is excreted by the kidneys. After this point there is slow clearance, with a biological half-life of 25 days. Body sites with high concentrations of lactoferrin cause normal uptake in the nasopharynx, bone marrow, spleen, and salivary and lacrimal glands. The critical organ is the colon, because of direct gastrointestinal secretion (Fig.10-1). Early images at 4 to 6 hours after injection are most useful for early detection of an intra-abdominal abscess. Total body scans are usually done at 24 to 48 hours. Colonic enemas are not consistently effective at clearing normal colonic activity and should not be routinely done. Accumulation of activity within the kidneys is common at 24 hours and may still be faintly seen at 48 hours. Breast uptake is commonly seen and may vary with the menstrual cycle. Transient lung uptake may be seen within the first 24 hours but tends

215

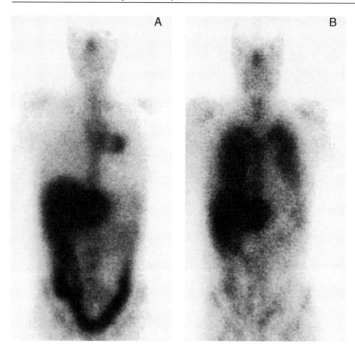

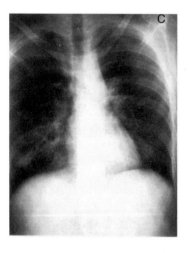

Figure 10-1. Prominent left hilar uptake in a patient with lymphoma. **(A)** Colonic activity is due primarily to direct gastrointestinal secretion of Ga67 **(B)** Bilateral symmetric lung uptake is seen on a follow-up examination and is due to interstitial pneumonitis secondary to bleomycin therapy. **(C)** Chest x-ray findings are minimal and reveal only nonspecific patchy bilateral basilar densities. **(D)** CT of the lung reveals subpleural consolidation, diffuse ground glass opacities, and interlobular septal thickening—all compatible with bleomycin toxicity.

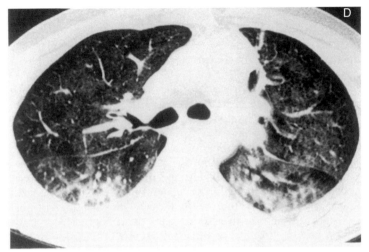

Figure 10-1. *continued*

to clear progressively. Recent lymphangiography may cause significantly increased pulmonary uptake. Normal uptake may be seen at noninfected surgical sites for 1 to 2 weeks.

Optimization of imaging is by use of a medium-energy collimator that can collimate the 300-keV photon. A slightly widened energy window of 30% is useful to increase the count rate so that 500,000 count images can be obtained. One million count images are preferable if there is a specific region of interest and sufficient patient cooperation. SPECT is most frequently employed for tumor imaging after a routine tumor imaging dose of 8 to 10 mCi is injected. SPECT is obtained using a 360-degree acquisition and is most useful for direct comparison with CT or MR imaging.

Although there are a high number of inflammatory processes that produce increased gallium activity, there are relatively few routine clinical applications of gallium scanning for inflammation or infection. There is an occasional role in the evaluation of the patient with **fever of unknown origin.** This is especially true in patients who have had a negative white blood cell study and whose symptoms have persisted for longer than 2 weeks.

Patients whose symptoms are more acute often benefit from a labeled leukocyte study, because results can be obtained quickly and the sensitivity of the two techniques is relatively similar. The great majority of patients with fever of unknown origin have a negative gallium study.

Gallium scanning is occasionally useful in the patient with **acquired immunodeficiency syndrome** (AIDS), since the sensitivity of gallium for *Pneumocystis carinii* infection is approximately 90%. Pneumocystis infection may be the initial presentation of AIDS, and the gallium scan may be positive in the setting of a normal chest radiograph. A normal gallium scan makes pneumocystis infection unlikely. Specificity of the gallium study is highest when there is diffuse bilateral pulmonary uptake with intensity greater than that of the liver. Pulmonary uptake equal to or greater than the liver is often described as grade 3 or grade 4 uptake. The finding of diffuse bilateral pulmonary uptake without lymph node involvement is most suggestive of pneumocystis infection. There are, however, some other causes of diffuse lung uptake, including **interstitial pneumonitis, drug toxicity,** and **cytomegalic virus infection.** When uptake is seen in an asymmetric pattern or a lobar pattern with hilar lymph node involvement, the findings are more suggestive of infection with *Mycobacterium avium intracellulare.* Uptake within nodes alone may be seen with lymphoma, and a combination of nodal and pulmonary uptake is most suggestive of an atypical infection. The generalized lymphadenopathy that is seen in patients with AIDS-related complex (ARC) is not thought to be gallium avid. Gallium uptake that is seen only within a lobe and without nodal involvement may be due to bacterial pneumonia. Uptake in multiple organs, including the lungs, eye, kidneys, and GI tract, is possible with CMV infection. A differentiating point of scintigraphy in the immunocompromised patient is that *Kaposi's sarcoma* is not gallium avid. **Sarcoidosis** is a cause of both increased pulmonary and lymph node gallium uptake. Drugs that cause increased pulmonary uptake alone include bleomycin and amiodarone.

Gallium scintigraphy may make a contribution in cases of suspected **osteomyelitis.** Three-phase bone scanning is usually adequate for diagnosis of uncomplicated osteomyelitis. When bone scan findings are questionable or there is a long-term complication of fracture or placement of orthopedic hardware, gallium may be helpful. Specifically, when gallium images are negative, there is a low likelihood of infection. When gallium images show uptake that is greater than that of Tc-99m-MDP or when the findings are not anatomically congruent, there is evidence for diagnosing osteomyelitis. For most applications In-111 granulo-cyte imaging combined with bone scanning is superior to gal-lium scintigraphy for diagnosing acute osteomyelitis. One notable exception is the significant role of gallium in the diagno-sis of vertebral osteomyelitis or **discitis.** Evidence suggests that gallium imaging is best for infection of the spine, because granu-locyte imaging has a low sensitivity for this application. Gal-lium-67 imaging is also useful for evaluating the activity of necrotizing external otitis of the temporal bone and the response to antibiotic therapy.

Gallium imaging is infrequently employed for infections below the diaphragm, where applications of CT, ultrasound, and In-111 leukocyte imaging are often more appropriate. Persistent renal or perirenal gallium accumulation more than 48 hours fol-lowing administration can suggest the presence of a **perinephric abscess** or **pyelonephritis.** False-positive causes of gallium uptake within the renal bed include obstruction, nephritis, rejection, amyloidosis, tumor, and acute tubular necrosis. Gallium accu-mulation within the renal bed or the small bowel or colon must always be viewed with caution because results may be variable. Studies are often most useful when there is no evidence of gal-lium accumulation.

A large number of tumors are gallium avid, and including **lung carcinoma, melanoma, hepatocellular carcinoma, soft-tis-sue sarcoma, testicular tumors, multiple myeloma, head** and **neck tumors, rhabdomyosarcoma,** and **neuroblastoma.** Unfortu-nately, the clinical application of gallium to study these tumors is controversial, and gallium imaging should be used only on a case-by-case basis. For instance, gallium scintigraphy is rarely useful for identifying occult metastases of lung cancer outside of the thorax. Gallium may occasionally be useful in differentiating the intense degree of uptake seen within a hepatoma from the lesser degree of uptake seen in a regenerating nodule. Recurrent gallium uptake within a head and neck tumor may indicate poor prognosis in a patient who has undergone therapy. Activity within the liver, spleen, and gastrointestinal tract makes imaging of abdominal and pelvic tumors difficult. Relatively higher-grade soft-tissue sarcomas tend to be quite gallium avid, although there is lower sensitivity for lesions involving the liver and the skeleton. There is reasonable sensitivity of gallium for melanoma, although sensitivity falls when lesions are smaller than 2 cm in diameter.

Gallium-67 imaging continues to be useful for the clinical management of **lymphoma,** because it provides input regarding staging, detection of relapse or progression, prediction of response to therapy, and prediction of outcome. The sensitivity for detection of **Hodgkin's disease** is at least 90%, and specificity may exceed that of CT and MRI. Tumor viability is usually correctly predicted when gallium uptake is seen within a residual soft-tissue mass noted by CT (Fig. 10-2). Sensitivity is highest for disease involving the mediastinal lymph nodes and superficial nodes and drops to approximately 50% for disease involving the periaortic or retroperitoneal nodes. Gallium scintigraphy is not a good predictor of splenic involvement by Hodgkin's lymphoma. The false-positive rate for gallium imaging in a patient with Hodgkin's lymphoma is approximately 5%.

Gallium is also an excellent choice for imaging of intermediate- or high-grade non-Hodgkin's lymphoma. There is a high gallium avidity for diffuse large-cell lymphomas, including diffuse histiocytic lymphoma and poorly differentiated lymphocytic lymphoma. There is also high gallium avidity for small non-cleaved cell lymphoma (Burkitt's lymphoma). Low-grade lymphomas such as the well-differentiated lymphocytic lymphoma have lower gallium avidity.

A major impact of gallium-67 is in predicting tumor viability when a residual mass is detected by CT (Fig. 10-3). A baseline study and sequential studies are most useful because gallium uptake may be slightly variable even for a specific tumor type. SPECT studies are useful for distinguishing normal gallium uptake within skeletal and soft-tissue structures and may provide a significant advantage over planar imaging when direct comparison is made with CT or MRI. Sequential studies are also necessary to document changing avidity of a tumor, the response of that tumor to therapy, and the timing of that therapeutic response. Sequential gallium images may also provide evidence of early effectiveness of therapy and therefore play a significant role in patient management.

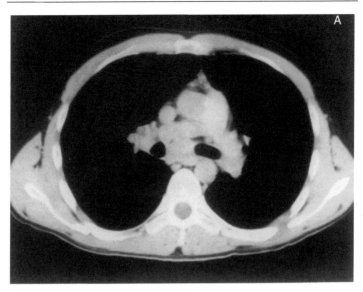

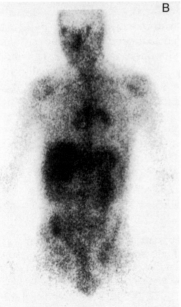

Figure 10-2. **(A)** Lung CT in a patient with Hodgkin's lymphoma reveals residual subcarinal and right and left hilar adenopathy following chemotherapy. **(B)** Anterior whole-body planar imaging 48 hours following intravenous administration of 10 mCi of Ga67 citrate reveals evidence of tumor viability within the residual mass noted by CT.

Labeled white blood cells now play a major role in the detection of infection and inflammation. *In-111 oxine* and In-111 tropolone can both be used to label cellular elements of the buffy coat. Thirty to 80 mL of whole blood are anticoagulated and allowed to sediment. A settling agent such as hydroxyethyl starch can be used to hasten the process. This results in a supernatant that is leukocyte rich but also contains many platelets and red blood cells (RBCs). The plasma is then centrifuged, and the white cell layer is incubated with 1 mCi of In-111 oxine for approximately 30 minutes. Oxine is the most commonly used agent for labeling and is a lipophilic agent that allows indium to enter the cell. Oxine then leaves the cell and the In-111 binds to intracellular proteins. The tropolone labeling method is investigational and has the advantage of allowing labeling of white cells in plasma. This is not possible for the oxine method, because indium binds the transferrin within plasma more avidly than the oxine. Labeling with 1 mCi of In-111 results in a dose of approximately 1500 rad to neutrophils, but this does not significantly alter phagocytic function. Lymphocytes receive a higher dose of approximately 9000 rad, which destroys the cells and therefore poses no threat from oncogenesis. The patient is given 500 µCi of In-111-labeled leukocytes intravenously and imaged with a medium-energy collimator using the 173- and 247-keV photopeaks (Fig. 10-4). An early image between 2 and 4 hours may be obtained, although the sensitivity is not as high as that at 24 hours. After injection there may be transient retention of the labeled cells within the lungs, but this usually clears by 24 hours. Splenic activity is highest at 24 hours, whereas liver and bone marrow show a lesser degree of uptake. There should be no activity within the renal or GI tract (Figure 10-5).

An alternative to In-111 labeling of leukocytes is the use of *Tc-99m-HMPAO*. HMPAO is a lipophilic agent used for cere-

Figure 10-3. **(A)** *Opposite page:* Prominent mediastinal adenopathy in a patient with Hodgkin's lymphoma. Forty-eight-hour gallium study reveals active disease within these sites corresponding to the chest x-ray findings. **(B)** Sensitivity is highest for disease involving mediastinal and superficial lymph nodes. **(C)** Following 2 months of therapy a follow-up chest x-ray reveals significant residual mediastinal soft-tissue mass. **(D)** Follow-up gallium study done during the same time period reveals resolution of mediastinal activity and strongly suggests early effectiveness of therapy.

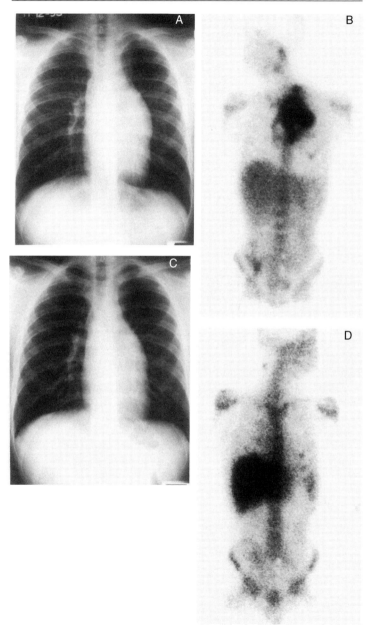

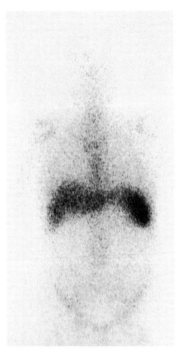

Figure 10-4. Anterior whole-body planar image 24 hours following intravenous injection of 500 μCi of indium-111-labeled leukocytes reveals no abnormal sites of activity. There is normal prominence of splenic activity and normal absence of gastrointestinal or genitourinary excretion.

bral perfusion imaging and changes into a secondary hydrophilic complex that binds primarily to mitochondria and the nucleus. Labeling can be done in plasma and shows a predilection for granulocytes. After injection there is initial uptake within the lungs, liver, and spleen followed by activity within the GU tract and bowel (Fig. 10-6). At 4 hours approximately 10% of patients show gallbladder activity, and at 24 hours colonic activity is the rule (Fig. 10-7). Tc-99m-HMPAO-labeled leukocytes may be preferable in patients in whom rapid diagnosis is needed, since images at 1 hour approach the sensitivity of the delayed images. Delayed images at 24 hours may be required in cases of more chronic infection. HMPAO-labeled leukocytes may also be the preferred agent for patients with an acute infection of the extremities or an infected vascular graft (Fig. 10-8).

There are a number of applications of In-111 leukocyte scanning, and these include the work-up of the patient with a clinical suspicion of abscess but no localizing signs. The lack of bowel

Figure 10-5. Anterior view of the abdomen 48 hours after injection of indium-111 leukocytes reveals normal intense activity within the spleen and faint diffuse activity within the colon. The patient had undergone colonic enema prior to examination. The findings suggest not a focal abscess or segment of inflamed bowel wall, but rather diffuse irritation of the colon.

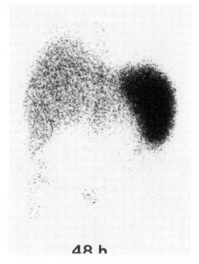

48 h

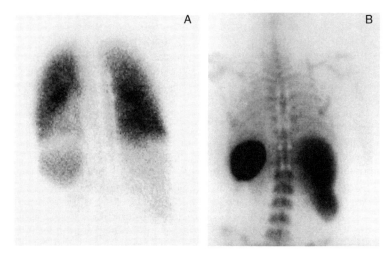

Figure 10-6. Posterior planar image obtained within 1 hour of injection of Tc99m-HMPAO-labeled leukocytes. **(A)** Early lung uptake is common and does not suggest the presence of infection. Twenty-four-hour posterior view of the same patient shows normal activity within the bone marrow liver and spleen and resolution of pulmonary uptake. **(B)** Harrington rods are present in the thoracolumbar region .

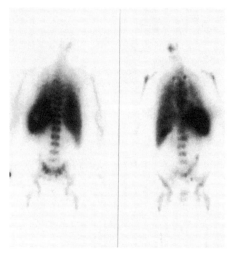

Figure 10-7. Posterior and anterior total body planar views 4 hours following intravenous injection of Tc99m-HMPAO-labeled leukocytes. There is normal transient pulmonary uptake. In approximately 10% of patients gallbladder activity is present, as is true in this case. A small amount of urinary excretion of a secondary complex is seen from a left-sided pelvic renal transplant.

excretion enhances the evaluation of the abdomen, where the sensitivity for intra-abdominal infection is greater than 90%. Patients with inflammatory bowel disease should be studied at 4 hours rather than at 24 hours because of possible shedding of labelled cells into the bowel lumen. The pattern of accumulation may suggest whether there is a focal abscess or a segment of inflamed bowel wall.

In-111-labeled leukocytes are occasionally useful for infections of the genitourinary tract. To avoid the high dose of indium-111 to the spleen, Tc-99m-HMPAO-labeled cells may be preferable in the pediatric population. Patients who are neutropenic may be studied adequately with donor leukocytes. Antibiotic therapy does not seem to have a significant effect on study sensitivity. Clinical experience has shown that the sensitivity of labeled leukocytes is insufficient for vertebral osteomyelitis and bacterial endocarditis. Causes of false-positive studies (Fig. 10–9) include gastrointestinal bleeding, swallowed labeled cells caused by endotracheal tubes, feeding tubes, pneumonia or sinusitis, inflamed intravenous catheter insertion sites, recent postoperative sites (Fig. 10-10), and colostomies or ileostomies.

Investigational new methods for evaluating the presence of inflammation or infection include the use of radioimmunoconjugates such as labeled murine monoclonal antigranulocyte anti-

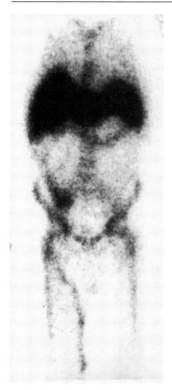

Figure 10-8.   Anterior planar view 24 hours following intravenous administration of Tc99m-HMPAO-labeled leukocytes reveals an infected right femoral–popliteal vascular graft. Normal colonic excretion is also present.

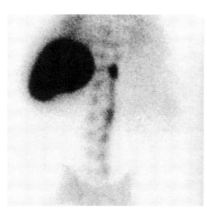

Figure 10-9.   Posterior view following administration of Tc99m-HMPAO-labeled leukocytes reveals uptake within the inferior vena cava due to the presence of extensive intravenous thrombus.

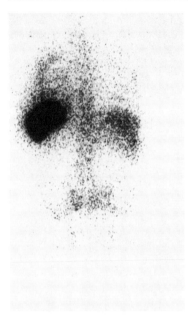

Figure 10-10. Posterior view obtained 24 hours after injection of 500 μCi of In-111 oxine-labeled leukocytes reveals normal splenic activity and increased activity within the left hemithorax. The positive finding is due to recent left-sided lung transplantation and multiple rib fractures.

bodies and labeled human polyclonal nonspecific IgG. The use of whole antibodies is complicated by the production of human antimouse antibodies in 10 to 40% of patients. Although sensitivity for infection appears to be high, specificity is limited because any inflammatory site may show uptake. A relatively recent surprising discovery was that nonspecific polyclonal IgG shows excellent sensitivity for bacterial and nonbacterial infections in human patients. Preparation involves In-111 DTPA chelation to IgG. Imaging is performed at 24 or 48 hours after injection of 1.5 mCi and shows biodistribution to the blood pool, liver, and spleen, with lesser activity in the kidneys, genitals, and nasopharynx. The dose to the spleen is somewhat less than that from In-111-labeled leukocytes. Proposed mechanisms for uptake include vascular permeability and binding to bacteria and Fc receptors on granulocytes. Advantages include the lack of handling of whole-blood products and the lack of production of human antimouse antibodies. Disadvantages include somewhat limited clinical experience and lower specificity for infection.

Other agents for imaging of infection include chemotactic peptides, which are a product of bacteria and stimulate chemotaxis.

Early results suggest that analogs of these peptides rapidly localize at infection sites. Tc-99m colloids have been advocated in the past for infection imaging because they are phagocytized by leukocytes.

A significant amount of research time and money has been spent on developing agents designed to be specific for imaging primary and metastatic cancer. Early developments concentrated on production of antibodies within laboratory animals such as rabbits, and this resulted in production of impure polyclonal antibodies, which gave nonspecific results. It was the description of the hybridoma antibody production technique in 1975 that allowed unlimited production of monoclonal antibodies with higher specificity. With this model lymphocytes are sensitized to an antigen and fused with mouse myeloma cells. The hybridoma produces antibodies by the method of the lymphocyte that benefits from the relative immortality of the myeloma cell.

The application of murine monoclonal antibodies has been hampered by the development of human antimouse antibodies (HAMA). Studies have also been limited by low target-to-background-activity ratios and cross reactivity with nonspecific antigens. The development of monoclonal antibodies has not completely solved the challenges associated with polyclonal antibodies. Significant visceral activity and high levels of activity within the liver and blood pool remain a problem. Nevertheless, a large number of monoclonal antibodies have been developed for imaging several types of tumors, including breast, melanoma, colorectal, prostate, and ovarian cancer. The radionuclide of choice has been indium-111 in most because since this avoids the problem of dehalogenation of iodine by the liver. The first FDA-approved monoclonal antibody was indium-111-labeled Mab B72.3, which localizes to tumor-associated antigen, a glycoprotein expressed by adenocarcinomas. After infusion of 5 mCi of In-111-labeled antibody, imaging is possible at 48 to 72 hours with reasonable sensitivity and specificity for ovarian and colorectal cancer. In general, monoclonal antibody imaging has occasionally been competitive with CT when tumor is present in the pelvis. CT is more sensitive for liver metastases. Larger injected doses of labeled antibody improve relative tumor uptake and serum half-life, but production of antiglobulin limits the number of repeated studies in humans. The relatively low immunogenicity of human rather than murine monocloncal antibodies makes them better candidates for future applications in cancer detection and therapy. Radiopharmaceutical costs will continue to seriously limit widespread clinical application of radiolabeled monoclonal antibodies.

A number of developments have taken place in the field of neuroendocrine scintigraphic imaging. Scintigraphic applications to abnormalities of the adrenal cortex and the adrenal medulla are possible. Disorders of the adrenal cortex may produce abnormalities in production of cortisol, aldosterone, or androgenic steroids. Disorders of the adrenal medulla may affect catecholamine levels. Occasionally, studies are performed with iodomethyl-19-norcholesterol, which functions as a precursor of adrenal corticosteroids. Patients are pretreated with Lugol's iodine and given 1 mCi per 1.7 m^2 of body surface area. Scanning begins at 48 hours and may continue for 5 days. When dexamethasone suppression is used the normal adrenal glands may not be visualized for 5 days. If suppression is used then symmetrical uptake suggests hyperplasia (which may be asymmetric in some cases), whereas unilateral uptake suggests the presence of adenoma. When suppression is not used, bilateral nonvisualization suggests the presence of adrenal carcinoma.

Imaging of the adrenal medulla is possible with metaiodobenzylguanidine (MIBG). This analog of guanethidine is taken up by an active amine transport mechanism and stored in presynaptic vesicles. Iodine-131-MIBG can be used to image neuroblastoma, ganglioneuroblastoma, paraganglioma, and pheochromocytoma. The primary work-up for pheochromocytoma involves biochemical tests and CT. Occasionally, MIBG is useful to localize extra-adrenal tumor sites. After a patient is pretreated with Lugol's solution, an intravenous dose of 0.5 mCi per 1.75 m^2 is given. Images may be obtained at 24, 48, and 72 hours after injection. Normal adrenal glands may be faintly seen, and normal sites of involvement include the liver, spleen, heart, and salivary glands on early images, and bladder and occasionally colon on later images.

Imaging of neuroendocrine tumors is now possible with the FDA-approved radiopharmaceutical *indium-111-pentetreotide* (OctreoScan). Pentetreotide is the DTPA conjugate of octreotide, which is an analog of somatostatin. Indium-111 pentetreotide binds to cell surface receptors for somatostatin and is indicated for imaging neuroendocrine tumors such as pheochromocytoma, neuroblastoma, medullary thyroid carcinoma, and carcinoid

(Fig. 10-11). Three mCi may be given for planar images and 6 mCi for SPECT imaging. Caution should be taken for patients who are being imaged for insulinoma in order to avoid hypoglycemia. Total body imaging is undertaken at 4 and 24 hours after injection. Scans should be obtained slowly for a total of approximately 500,000 counts in order to obtain sufficient count density. Scans at 48 hours may be necessary to differentiate bowel accumulation from tumor activity (Fig. 10-12). Somatostatin receptor imaging with In-111 pentetreotide is now beginning to replace the use of iodine-131 MIBG for imaging of neuroendocrine tumors.

Thallium-201 has been useful for differentiating intermediate and high-grade lymphomas of the brain from sites of infection. Clinical experience has not been sufficient to seriously test the specificity of this finding. Applications of thallium-201 to bone, lung, and breast cancer have not found widespread acceptance.

Figure 10-11. Posterior and anterior images of the thorax and abdomen 24 hours after intravenous injection of 3 mCi of indium-111 pentetreotide (OctreoScan). Normal gastrointestinal, renal, and thyroid activity is present. Pituitary uptake may also be seen commonly on many studies. Abnormal focus of right hilar activity is due to an intrabronchial carcinoid tumor.

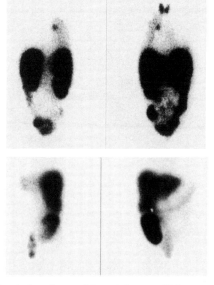

Figure 10-12. Posterior and anterior views of the abdomen 48 hours after intravenous administration of 3 mCi of In-111-pentetreotide (OctreoScan). Scans at 48 hours may be useful to differentiate bowel accumulation from tumor activity. In this case right lower quadrant uptake is due to presence of a right-sided renal transplant.

Thallium-201 is taken up by Kaposi's sarcoma when a gallium-67 study is negative. Thallium-201 imaging is possible for thyroid cancer while a patient is receiving synthroid for suppression. Unfortunately, thallium-201 does not predict which patients can be successfully treated with iodine-131 therapy.

Recent clinical experience suggests that *Tc-99m-sestamibi* may be useful in a select group of patients with suspected breast cancer. A negative study seems to have an excellent predictive value in ruling out the presence of cancer (Fig. 10-13). The specificity of a positive study is somewhat limited. Twenty mCi of Tc-99m-sestamibi are injected intravenously into the arm contralateral to the breast with suspected pathology. A 10-minute lateral image of the breast is then obtained 5 minutes after injection in either the upright or prone position. A 30-degree posterior oblique image may be obtained if an abnormal site of uptake is seen near the chest wall. A 10-minute lateral image is then repeated 1 hour after injection followed by a 10-minute anterior image done with the arms raised. Prone imaging provides the advantage of better separation of breast tissue from the

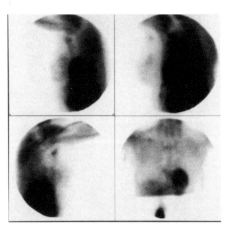

Figure 10-13. Breast imaging obtained 10 minutes after the intravenous injection of 20 mCi of Tc99m sestamibi in the left lateral and left posterior oblique (top row) and right lateral and anterior (bottom row) orientations. There was no significant focal sestamibi accumulation to correlate with a mammographic abnormality. Prone imaging done with a specially designed imaging table can be useful to separate intense skeletal muscle uptake from breast tissue. Normal myocardial activity is seen in the anterior projection.

pectoralis muscle and liver but requires a specially designed table. The exact cellular mechanism of sestamibi uptake by breast cancer is unknown, although mitochondrial density may play a role. Scintigraphic imaging with sestamibi is not indicated as a replacement for screening mammography.

A promising area of imaging for oncology is the use of fluorine-18 fluorodeoxyglucose (FDG), also known as *F-18 fludeoxyglucose*. The elevated rate of glycolysis in tumor tissue causes uptake of F-18 FDG into tumor cells, where it is phosphorylated by hexokinase and trapped. The 110-minute half-life of fluorine-18 allows imaging by PET and SPECT. The initial application of F-18 FDG PET was to the evaluation of neurologic disorders, including seizure, dementia, and neoplasm. Images of high resolution and high specificity were also obtained when F-18 FDG was applied to cardiac PET imaging. The most recent application has been to oncologic imaging, where F-18 FDG provides images of high target-to-background ratio. FDG uptake has been described in **tumors of the brain, oropharynx, thyroid, breast, lung** (Fig. 10-14), **colon** and **rectum, genitourinary system, bone,** and **soft tissues,** as well as in **lymphoma** and **malignant melanoma.** Large field-of-view, high-sensitivity scanners have now made whole-body PET scanning possible within a 60-minute period. Patients are typically injected intravenously with a dose of approximately 10 mCi of F-18 FDG, and tomographic studies are obtained in the axial, coronal, and sagittal plains. Because relatively prominent FDG accumulation occurs in only a few normal sites (e.g., brain, myocardium, and renal pelvis and bladder), there is relatively prominent accumulation of FDG at tumor sites, producing a study of high sensitivity and acceptable specificity. Possible false-positive findings include sites of inflammation or infection and occasionally the gastrointestinal tract. A false-negative result could occur if a metastatic lesion was of very small diameter (perhaps less than 3 mm) or if a metastasis was present within a site of normally high FDG uptake. Recent studies show considerable promise in staging malignant melanoma and detecting the presence or absence of axillary adenopathy in patients with breast cancer. Because protein synthesis may also be elevated in tumor tissue there is ongoing experimental investigation of C-11 labeled amino acids such as methionine, tyrosine, and thymidine for use in oncologic imaging. Clinical experience has not yet established a role for these new agents.

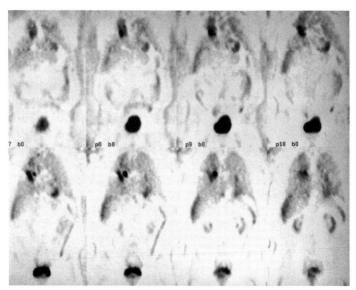

Figure 10-14. Serial coronal PET images of the thorax and abdomen following intravenous injection with approximately 10 mCi of F18 FDG. This 63-year-old male smoker developed a lung nodule on serial chest radiographs. The F18 FDG PET study reveals intense uptake within the right-sided nodule and a metastatic focus within the ipsilateral hilum. Since the metastasis was on the same side of the mediastinum as the primary the patient was taken to surgery. Surgery confirmed the PET finding. (Image courtesy of Donald S. Schauwecker, Ph.D., M.D.)

The major limitations of PET involve the high cost of construction, maintenance, and operation, and the unavailability of this relatively new modality. A development which is under investigation is the use of SPECT gamma camera systems equipped with ultra-high-energy collimators for the 511-keV energy spectrum. Electronics are being modified to take maximum advantage of the relatively high signal of the 511-keV photon and the simultaneous 180-degree photon emissions. These ultra-high-energy collimators have a core length of approximately 80 mm with a 4-mm-diameter hole and 2.5-mm septal thickness. Each collimator weighs approximately 142 kg, which is supportable by dual-headed camera systems. The energy window is around 511 keV ± 10%. Because of high F-18 FDG tumor-to-background ratios of 3:1 to

10:1, there is good sensitivity of these SPECT systems for viable tumors larger than 2–3 cm in diameter. PET continues to be the preferred modality for F-18 FDG imaging when smaller lesions are being targeted. A remaining challenge is the rapid delivery of radiopharmaceutical to various imaging sites, which is made difficult by the short 110-minute half-life of fluorine-18 and the limited number of production centers.

An additional role for nuclear medicine in oncology is the use of *P-32 chromic phosphate colloid* for intraperitoneal treatment of **disseminated ovarian cancer.**The goal of treatment is to distribute P-32 chromic phosphate throughout the peritoneal cavity in a distribution that is similar to the expected spread of ovarian carcinoma cells. A catheter is placed into the peritoneum under sterile technique and Tc-99m-sulfur colloid is instilled with at least 250 to 500 mL of saline to assess distribution throughout the peritoneal cavity (Figs. 10-15 and 10-16). Ten to 15 mCi of P-32 chromic phosphate are then instilled into the peritoneum and flushed with additional saline. P-32 is a pure beta emitter with a half-life of 14.3 days and a mean beta energy of 695 keV. The average penetration of the beta particles is 3 mm into soft tissue, and the approximate dose to the peritoneum for every 10 mCi is 6000 rad. Patients have been given up to 42 mCi of P-32 in divided weekly doses without developing serious complications. There is evidence that P-32 enhances cisplatin and carboplatin killing of cell lines of disseminated intraperitoneal ovarian carcinoma. Other applications of colloidal P-32 include treatment of cystic cranial neoplasms such as **craniopharyngioma** and the treatment of **intracavitary fluid collections** of the pleura or pericardium. P-32 chromic phosphate may also be instilled into the knee or elbow joint in patients with **hemophilic arthropathy** and **chronic joint effusions**. The recommended dose of P-32 for synovectomy is approximately 1 mCi for the knee joint and 0.5 mCi for the elbow joint.

P-32 has also been used in the form of intravenous P-32 sodium phosphate for **polycythemia vera.** Patients who are not controlled by phlebotomy or chemotherapy may benefit from intravenous administration of 2.3 mCi of P-32 sodium phosphate per square meter of body surface area. If necessary, patients may be retreated 3 months later with a dose that is 25% greater than the initial dose but no greater than 7 mCi. Dose to the skeleton is approximately 315 rad for every 5 mCi of P-32.

Figure 10-15. Peritoneal distribution study after intraperitoneal instillation of 5 mCi of Tc99m sulfur colloid and 250 to 500 mL of saline. The patient should be encouraged to shift into both decubitus positions several times prior to imaging in order to assess potential distribution of intraperitoneal P32 chromic phosphate for treatment of intraperitoneal spread of ovarian cancer. This study shows normal intraperitoneal distribution of sulfur colloid with complete outline of the peritoneum.

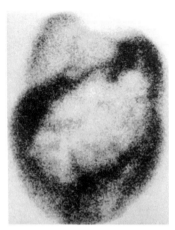

Figure 10-16. Intraperitoneal flow distribution study done after instillation of Tc-99m-sulfur colloid and saline reveals a photopenic defect in the left lower quadrant that corresponds to peritoneal tumor deposit by CT. Comparison of this type of peritoneal distribution study with peritoneally enhanced CT show good correlation. This patient received intraperitoneal P32 therapy because distribution of sulfur colloid was thought to be adequate.

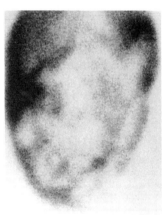

Suggested Reading

Bonnin F, Lumbroso J, Tenenbaum F, et al. Refining interpretation of MIBG scans in children. *J Nucl Med* 1994;35:803-810.

Conti PS, Keppler JS, Halls JM. Positron emission tomography: a financial and operational analysis *AJR* 1994;162:1279-1286.

Corstens FHM, Oyen WJG and Becker WS. Radioimmunocojugates in the detection of infection and inflammation. *Semin Nucl Med* 1993;13(2):148-164.

Datz FL: The current status of radionuclide infection imaging. In Freeman LM, ed.: *Nuclear Medicine Annual.* New York:Raven Press, 1993.

Datz FL: Indium-111-labeled leukocytes for the detection of infection: current status. *Semin Nucl Med* 1994;24(2):92-109.

De Jager R, Abdel-Nabi H, Serafini A, Pecking A, Klein J and Hanna Jr. M. Current status of cancer immunodetection with radiolabeled human monoclonal antibodies. *Semin Nucl Med* 1993;23(2):165-179.

Drane WE, Abbott FD, Nicole MW, Mastin ST, Kuperus JH. Technology for FDG SPECT with a relatively inexpensive gamma camera. *Radiology* 1994;191:461-465.

Fischman AJ, Rubin RH, Khaw BA, et al: Detection of acute inflammation with 111-In-labeled nonspecific polyclonal IgG. *Semin Nucl Med* 1988;18:335-344.

Front D, Ben-Haim S, Israel O, et al. Lymphoma: Predictive value of Ga-67 scintigraphy after treatment. *Radiology* 1992;182:359-363.

Front D and Israel O. The role of Ga-67 scintigraphy in evaluating the results of therapy of lymphoma patients. *Semin Nucl Med* 1995;25(1):60-71.

Gloviczki P, Calcagno D, Schirger A. Noninvasive evaluation of the swollen extremity: experiences with 190 lymphoscintigraphic examinations. *Vasc Surg* 1989;9(5):683-690.

Gupta NC and Prezio JA: Radionuclide imaging in osteomyelitis. *Semin Nucl Med* 1988;18(4):287-299.

Jamar F, Fiasse R, Leners N, Pauwels S. Somatostatin receptor imaging with indium-111-pentetreotide in gastroenteropancreatic neuroendocrine tumors: safety, efficacy and impact on patient management. *J Nucl Med* 1995;36:542-549.

Keenan AM. Immunolymphoscintigraphy. *Semin Nucl Med* 1989;19:322-331.

Khalkhali I, Mena I, Jouranne E, et al. Prone scintimammography in patients with suspicion of carcinoma of the breast. *J Am Coll Surg* 1994;78:491-497.

Krenning EP, Kwekkeboom DJ, Bakker WH. Somatostatin receptor scintigraphy with [^{111}In-DTPA-D-Phe^1]- and [^{123}I-Tyr^3]-octreotide: the Rotterdam experience with more than 1000 patients. *Eur J Nucl Med* 1993;20:716-731.

Lamberts SWJ, Bakker WH, et al. Somatostatin-receptor imaging in the localization of endocrine tumors. *N Engl J Med* 1990;323:1246-1249.

Lee JD, Kim DI, Lee JT, Chang JW and Park CY. Indium-111-pentetreotide imaging in intra-axial brain tumors: comparison with thallium-201 SPECT and MRI. *J Nucl Med* 1995;36:537-541.

Martin WH, Delbeke D, Patton JA, Sandler MP. Detection of malignancies with SPECT versus PET, with 2-[fluorine-18] fluoro-2-deoxy-D-glucose. *Radiology* 1996;198:225-231.

Martin WH, Delbeke D, Patton JA, et al. FDG-SPECT: correlation with FDG-PET. *J Nucl Med* 1995;36:988-995.

Miller RF: Nuclear medicine and AIDS. *Eur J Nucl Med* 1990;16:103-118.

Okada J, Yoshikawa K, Itami M, et al. Positron emission tomography using fluorine-18-fluorodeoxyglucose in malignant lymphoma: a comparison with proliferative activity. *J Nucl Med* 1992;33:325-329.

Palestro CJ: The current role of gallium imaging in infection. *Semin Nucl Med* 1994; 24:128-141.

Pattillo RA, Collier BD, Abdel-Dayem H, et al. Phosphorus-32-chromic phosphate for ovarian cancer: I. Fractionated low-dose intraperitoneal treatments in conjunction with platinum analog chemotherapy. *J Nucl Med* 1995;36:29-36.

Podoloff DA, Patt YZ, Curley SA, Kim EE, Bhadkamkar VA. Imaging of colorectal carcinoma with technetium-99m radiolabeled Fab fragments. *Semin Nucl Med* 1993;23(2):89-98.

Ruiz A, Ganz WI, Post JD, et al. Use of thallium-201 brain SPECT to differentiate cerebral lymphoma for toxoplasma encephalitis in AIDS patients. *Am J Neuroradiol* 1994;15:1885-1894.

Schauwecker DS: The scintigraphic diagnosis of osteomyelitis. *AJR* 1992;158:9-18.

Siegel HJ, Luck JV Jr , Siegel ME, Quines C, Anderson E. Hemarthrosis and synovitis associated with hemophilia: clinical use of P-32 chromic phosphate synoviorthesis for treatment. *Radiology* 1994;190:257-261.

Steinert HC, Huch Boni RA, Buck A, et al. Malignant melanoma: staging with whole-body positron emission tomography and 2-[F-18]-fluoro-2-deoxy-D-glucose. *Radiology* 1995;195:705-709.

Strauss LG, Conti PS. The applications of PET in clinical oncology. *J Nucl Med* 1991;32:623-648.

Uren RF, Howman-Giles RB, Shaw HM, Thompson JF, McCarthy WH. Lymphoscintigraphy in high-risk melanoma of the trunk: predicting draining node groups, defining lymphatic channels and locating the sentinel node. *J Nucl Med* 1993;34:1435-1440.

Van Lingen A, Juijgens PC, Visser FC, et al. Performance characteristics of a 511-keV collimator for imaging positron emitters with a standard gamma camera. *Eur J Nucl Med* 1992;19:315-321.

Waxman AD, Ramanna L, Memsic LD, et al. Thallium scintigraphy in the evaluation of mass abnormalities of the breast. *J Nucl Med* 1993; 34:18-23.

Chapter 11

Physics, Instrumentation, and Radiochemistry

Radioactivity

Nuclear medicine imaging is frequently performed with radio-pharmaceuticals consisting of organ-specific pharmaceuticals labeled with radioactive isotopes. Occasionally, the isotopes are used without a separate pharmaceutical; the isotope is then the radiopharmaceutical. The radioactivity of all radioisotopes decays exponentially. The rate of this physical decay is expressed in terms of the half-life ($T_{1/2}$), which is the time required for the radioactivity to decrease by one-half. The activity A_t at time t is then

$$A_t = A_0 \left(\tfrac{1}{2}\right)^{\frac{t}{T_{1/2}}}$$

where A_o is the starting radioactivity.

If a 10-mCi dose of I-131 is on hand at 9 A.M. for a patient who fails to arrive until the next morning at 9 A.M., this formula can be used to calculate the dose the patient will actually receive.

A_0 = 10 mCi
$T_{1/2}$ = 8 days
t = 1 day
A_t = 10 $\left(\tfrac{1}{2}\right)^{1/8}$ = 9.17 mCi

The effective half-life of a radiopharmaceutical's radioactivity in the body is less than the physical half-life of the isotope because the radiopharmaceutical is eliminated from the body. The half-life of this elimination process is called the biological half-life. These quantities are related as follows:

$$T_e = \frac{T_{1/2}\, T_B}{T_{1/2} + T_B}$$

where T_e = effective half-life, $T_{1/2}$ = physical half-life, and T_B = biological half-life. For example, if the half-life of iodine in the thyroid is 60 days, then the effective half-life is

$$T_e = \frac{(8)(60)}{8 + 60} = 7.06 \text{ days}$$

Radioactive Decay

Radioactivity occurs when an element's unstable nuclei undergo transitions that result in increased stability of the nuclei. The intensity of radioactivity is related to the number of nuclear transitions per second. Two systems of units are in use. The becquerel (Bq) is one nuclear transition per second, and the curie (Ci) represents 3.7×10^{10} nuclear transitions per second.

1 Ci = 3.7×10^{10} Bq
1 mCi = 37 MBq
1 MBq = 27 μCi

Medically important radionuclides decay by four mechanisms: beta emission, positron emission, electron capture, and isomeric transition. These processes are characterized by the changes that occur in the number of neutrons *(N)* and the number of protons *(Z)*. The atomic mass number *(A)* is the sum of N and Z. An element X is symbolized as

$$^A_Z X$$

Medical radioisotopes are often designated as X-*A* (e.g., I-123).

The term *element* implies characterization of a substance by its atomic number. The term *nuclide* implies characterization by both Z and N; thus there are many more nuclides than elements. *Radionuclides* are radioactive nuclides.

Isotopes are variations of an element that contain different numbers of neutrons but the same number of protons. Only some isotopes are radioactive, and they are radioisotopes.

Isobars are nuclides that have the same total number of neutrons and protons but different atomic numbers. Isobars cannot be the same element, whereas isotopes are always of the same element.

Isomers are nuclides that have the same numbers of neutrons and protons but different nuclear energy levels. Isomers are always the same element. Isotones are nuclides that have the same number of neutrons.

The nuclear transitions that produce radioactivity are isobaric and isomeric. Nuclides with equal or approximately equal numbers of neutrons and protons tend to be stable, whereas nuclides with significant differences in these numbers tend to be unstable and therefore radioactive. Transitions that result in isobaric transitions to a stable state are beta emission, positron emission, and electron capture. Nuclides that contain a neutron-to-proton ratio that is too high for stability undergo transition by the conversion of a neutron into a proton with the accompanying emission of an electron that in this setting is called a beta particle. This process reduces the neutron-to-proton ratio and increases stability.

If the ratio of neutrons to protons is too low for stability, two kinds of transition can take place. In positron emission, a proton is converted into a neutron with accompanying emission of a positron, which is an atomic particle having the mass of an electron but a positive rather than a negative charge. Soon after its emission, this positron interacts with a nearby electron and both particles are annihilated. This annihilation is accompanied by the radiation of two photons, each with an energy of 511 keV. These photons leave the site of annihilation in opposite directions, a fact that is useful in medical PET (positron emission tomography) imaging.

The second mechanism by which a low neutron-to-proton ratio can be corrected is electron capture. In this process an electron in an inner shell reacts with a nuclear proton to produce a neutron. The accompanying radiation is the result of shifts in the orbits of the remaining electrons and may be either characteristic x-ray photons or Auger electrons. The characteristic x-radiation is what makes these nuclides useful in medical imaging.

Following isobaric transition, most nuclides remain in an unstable state and undergo isomeric transition to produce the stable daughter state. This final process of stabilization may occur in one or several steps, each of which is associated with the emission of a gamma photon. Gamma photons have zero mass and an energy that is characteristic of the nuclide. Alternately, the excess nuclear energy can be transferred to one of the atom's electrons. This transfer of energy causes the electron to leave the atom, with resulting shifts in the orbits occupied by the remaining electrons. This shift results in the radiation of characteristic x-rays or Auger electrons as in electron capture. The isomeric transition usually occurs immediately after the isobaric transition. When the isomeric transmission occurs after a delay, the state of the nucleus before the isomeric transmission takes place is called a metastable state. The metastable state is desirable in medical imaging because the isobaric transition that occurs before the metastable state is associated with radiation that contributes to patient dose but is useless for imaging. Nuclides that have already undergone the isobaric transition radiate only gamma photons, the radiation that is useful for imaging. Technetium-99m (Tc-99m) is a metastable nuclide derived from the isobaric transition of molybdenum. The metastable state is indicated by the *m* following the mass number 99.

Nuclear transition in some nuclides is accompanied by alpha radiation. Each alpha particle consists of two protons and two neutrons. Alpha particles travel only very short distances and are therefore useless for medical imaging. Radium is an alpha emitter that can be used therapeutically. When radium, usually in the form of small needles, is inserted into tissue, the tissue immediately surrounding the needles receives a very high dose of radiation, but distant tissue receives essentially no radiation.

Certain medically useful radionuclides, notably Tc-99m, can be produced locally in generators. The generator contains an exchange column to which is firmly bound the parent element (e.g., Mo-99) of the desired daughter radionuclide (e.g., Tc-99m). After the parent nuclide undergoes isobaric transition, a new element is formed and has altered chemical properties from the parent. Because of this chemical change, the daughter nuclide is not firmly bound to the column and can be washed off with saline. If the half-life of the parent nuclide is a few times that of the daughter nuclide, a state of transient equilibrium between the parent and daughter radioactivities is approached. In this state, the ratio of radioactivities of the parent and daughter nuclides remains constant as the nuclides decay. Isotopes other than Tc-99m that can be produced in generators are indium-113m and strontium-89m. Table 11-1 summarizes the mechanisms of nuclear transitions.

Instrumentation

Gamma Camera

Nuclear medicine images are formed in a system in which radioactivity from the patient is converted into light by a scintillation crystal. This light is insufficiently bright to form photographic images directly, so it is first detected by very sensitive photo multiplier tubes (PM tubes) and then electronically amplified. The scintillation crystal is a plate about 1 cm thick. If the crystal were placed close to a patient to whom a radiopharmaceutical had been administered, a useful light image would not be generated, because radiation impinging on the crystal comes from all directions and locations in the patient. This problem is overcome through the use of collimators. In the parallel hole design, many parallel lead-walled tubes (holes) are placed between the crystal and the patient. The holes prevent radiation that does not come from a direction perpendicular to the crystal from striking the crystal. The holes need not be parallel but can converge or diverge from the crystal, resulting in magnification or minifica-

Table 11–1. Common transitions in nuclear medicine isotopes. Gamma radiation can occur in both electron capture and isomeric transition. Both gamma and x-ray radiation, which are identical except for their sources, can occur in electron capture. e^- = election; e^+ = positron; ν = nutrino; $\bar{\nu}$ = antinutrino; γ = gamma particle; $\times$ = x-ray; m = metastable.

Transition	General Formula	Examples
isobaric: beta emission	$^A_Z X \rightarrow ^A_{z+1}Y + e^- + \bar{\nu}$	$^{99}_{42}Mo \rightarrow ^{99m}_{43}Tc + e^- + \bar{\nu}$
isobaric: positron emission	$^A_Z X \rightarrow ^A_{z-1}Y + e^+ + \nu$	$^{18}_9 F \rightarrow ^{18}_8 O + e^+ + \bar{\nu}$
isobaric: electron capture	$^A_Z X + \text{orbital } e^- \rightarrow ^A_{z+1}Y + \nu$	$^{111}_{49}In + \text{orbital } e^- \xrightarrow{\gamma} ^{111}_{48}Cd + \nu$ $^{201}_{81}Tl + \text{orbital } e^- \xrightarrow{\chi} ^{201}_{80}Hg + \nu$
isomeric	$^A_Z X \xrightarrow{\gamma} ^A_Z Y$	$^{99m}_{43}Tc \xrightarrow{\gamma} ^{99}_4 Tc$

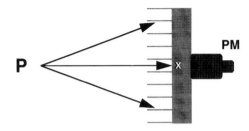

Figure 11–1. Arrangement of collimator, crystal, and photomultiplier tubes. Gamma particles originating from point *P* impinge on the crystal, causing scintillation at point *X*. The resulting light is detected by the photomultiplier tube PM. Septa in the collimator prevent off-axis photons from reaching the collimator.

tion of the image. The light image formed in the crystal is converted into an electronic signal by the multiple PM tubes on the side of the crystal opposite the collimator. Multiple tubes (rather than only one) are used to allow for the electronic localization of scintillation events in the crystal (Figs. 11–1, 11–2).

Collimator design involves a compromise of sensitivity, image resolution, and rejection of scattered radiation. Thick lead walls of the collimator holes reduce image degradation caused by scatter that penetrates the walls but reduces system sensitivity by obscuring more of the crystal. Large holes increase sensitivity by reducing the percentage of the crystal that is obscured by the walls but reduce image resolution because more oblique photon pathways are open to each crystal location. Several collimator designs are available that reflect different choices in these trade-offs. The designs are usually specified by their intended energy (higher energies require thicker walls) and by their relative sensitivity.

The pinhole collimator has only a single hole in a lead baffle that is mounted several inches from the crystal. In this design the single hole causes an image to be formed in the crystal analogous to the formation of an image in a photographic camera by the lens. As the hole size is increased sensitivity increases but image resolution decreases. Pinhole collimators can be designed for high resolution but have low sensitivity. The size of the projected image in the crystal changes as an organ's distance from

information about the photons striking the crystal and so can be used to differentiate direct radiation from an organ of interest from lower-energy scattered radiation that degrades the image. The camera contains a pulse height analyzer (PHA) that can be set to accept energy levels only within a specified range.

Each scintillation can be localized by the system, which recognizes the scintillation as the simultaneous detection of the light pulse by several nearby PM tubes. Once the system has identified the scintillation by this coincidence technique, the location of the scintillation is computed from the relative electrical intensities in PM tubes at known locations.

Computer and Digital Processing

The electrical signals from the PM tubes are continuously variable (analog). Similarly, the electrical signals sent to the cathode ray tube that is directly viewed or photographed are analog. Most nuclear medicine images are altered in some way before being viewed or filmed, and this image processing is done by a digital computer. The analog PM tube output signals must therefore be converted to digital form and the computer output must be converted to analog form. Within the computer each image is represented as a patchwork of tiny areas, each of which is associated with a number that corresponds to the intensity of a corresponding picture element (pixel) in the image. The image formats are frequently square, and the images contain 64×64, 128×128, or 256×256 pixels corresponding to 4096, 16,384, and 65,536 pixels, respectively, in each of the three formats. Computers represent numbers in a binary (base 2) system; the digits of each binary number are represented in the computer as bits. By convention, 1 byte equals 8 bits. Nuclear medicine image pixel intensities are frequently represented as 8-, 12-, or 16-bit numbers. The number of possible values represented by n bits is 2 raised to the nth power. Therefore a pixel intensity represented by 8 bits can have 256 possible brightnesses (gray-scale levels).

Among the operations performed by the computer on pixels and images are smoothing, background subtraction, and electrocardiogram (ECG) gating. Smoothing operations replace a pixel's value with an average of its value and the values of its neighbors. The result is that sudden changes in pixel intensity from one pixel to the next are reduced, partially eliminating the random statistical variation in pixel intensities. This random variation is one form of image noise and is particularly trouble-some in low-count images.

The organ of interest in a nuclear medicine image is usually partially obscured by an overlay of radioactivity coming from structures other than the organ. This situation can be partially corrected by background subtraction, a process in which a value roughly corresponding to the background intensity is subtracted from each pixel in the image.

In gated blood pool cardiac imaging serial images, perhaps 16, are acquired through a single cardiac cycle. Because the resulting count totals in each image are too low to form useful images, this process is repeated for several hundred cardiac cycles until each of the 16 images is represented by enough radioactive counts to form a usable image. The acquisition of the repeated 16-image series is synchronized with the cardiac cycle by the computer and an associated ECG system.

The ways in which data received by the computer from the camera are formatted into images are known as acquisition modes. In frame mode acquisition, the pixels of an image are represented as specific addresses in the computer memory before acquisition starts. Each scintillation in the camera crystal results in a count being added to the memory address of the pixel corresponding to the crystal location in which the scintillation occurred. In list mode acquisition, each scintillation is associated with its own memory address. A disadvantage of list mode acquisition is that it requires more computer memory than frame mode acquisition. List mode acquisition, however, can be faster than frame mode. The way in which the stored list mode data are used to form an image is at the discretion of the computer operator. For example, acquired counts during a gated blood pool study that are later determined to have been acquired during arrhythmias can be excluded from the final image sequence. This exclusion would be impossible in frame mode acquisition because information about the exact sequence of scintillations would have been lost.

Image Quality

Nuclear medicine image quality can be described in terms of contrast, resolution, and noise. Contrast is the difference in image intensity corresponding to differences in radioactivity in the patient. In general, high contrast is desirable, as between a bone metastasis and surrounding normal bone in a bone scan.

Contrast can be adversely affected by radiation from tissues surrounding the organ of interest or by scattered radiation. The effect of scattered radiation can be controlled by the image acquisition hardware in two ways. First, the pulse height analyzer window is set narrow enough to include primary radiation energies but exclude lower scatter energies. Second, scattered photons can be eliminated from the image to the degree that the collimator intercepts them because of their random directions.

Resolution, measured in lines per centimeter, is a measure of the clarity of the images that the system produces. Resolution is tested by placing strips of lead on the camera face (with or without a collimator in place) and exposing the camera to a diffuse source of radiation (flood source). The width of the lead strips is kept equal to their separation, and separation is made smaller and smaller until the alternating strips of high and low intensity in the image are just barely discernible; the resolution is then expressed in lines/per centimeter, corresponding to the number of lead strips per centimeter. In practice, the lead strips are mounted in a resolution phantom, which is a fixture that contains several groups of strips; these groups have different strip widths and are imaged simultaneously (Fig. 11–3). Alternately, resolution can be measured by imaging a small radioactive point or line and plotting the image intensity as a function of distance from the center of the source. If the distance between positions on each side of the maximum of this function are measured where the function is one-half of its maximum value, the result in millimeters is the full width at half maximum (FWHM). The function is called the point spread function or line spread function, depending on whether a point or line source is used. FWHM is the reciprocal of resolution, so a typical system having an FWHM of 0.8 cm will have a resolution of 1.25 lines/cm.

Blur is the term used to refer to imperfect resolution. The important contributors to blur are patient motion, intrinsic camera blur, and collimator blur. Camera blur can be reduced through the use of a thin crystal; however, this choice results in low camera sensitivity. A high number of PM tubes in the camera can reduce blur but increases expense. Collimator blur is reduced by reducing hole size and increasing hole length, but these factors reduce sensitivity. Collimator design is thus a compromise, and designs are generally categorized as high resolution, general purpose, or high sensitivity.

Image noise is distracting information that is different from the

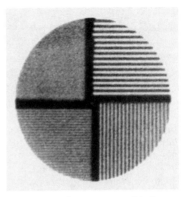

Figure 11–3. Resolution test. The phantom used to generate this image was placed between a flood source and the camera. The lead bar widths are 0.25 inch (upper right), 0.188 inch (lower right), 0.125 inch (lower left), and 0.083 inch (upper left). The smallest resolvable bars in this test were 0.125 inch in width. Since the separators between the lead strips are also 0.125 inch wide, there are four strips per inch, corresponding to a resolution of four lines per inch (1.57 lines per centimeter) and a FWHM of 0.25 inch (0.64 cm).

desired information. The main cause of noise in nuclear medicine images is statistical variation in count density among locations in the image. This noise results from the relatively low number of scintillations that produce an image. Statistical noise can be improved to a degree by image smoothing, also known as lowpass filtering, but this process also degrades the desired information somewhat.

Two other sources of image degradation are nonuniformity and spatial distortion. Nonuniformity is caused by inequality among the PM tube outputs. Uniformity can be tested with a flood source placed near the camera crystal or by the use of a point source placed several feet from the noncollimated camera face (Figs. 11–4 to 11–6). Spatial distortion results from errors in the system's calculation of the locations of sources in the patient. Spatial distortion can be tested by imaging phantoms of known geometric dimensions.

Single Photon Emission Computed Tomography

Most single photon emission computed tomography (SPECT) is carried out with a standard gamma camera that rotates around

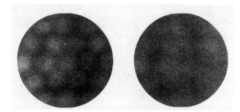

Figure 11–4. Off-peak nonuniformity. When the camera energy acceptance window is not centered on the energy peak of the imaged isotope, nonuniformity results. The pattern of nonuniformity is not always predictable; in this case, the image on the left was obtained from a flood source with the energy window set above the peak, and the image at the right was obtained with the window set below the peak.

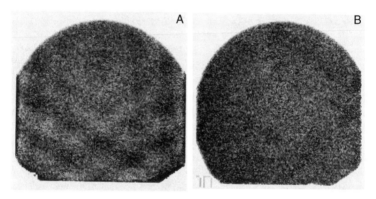

Figure 11–5. Nonuniformity due to PM tube imbalance. Most cameras provide for automatic balancing of the PM tubes. **(A)** The PM tubes are not balanced. Following the PM tube balancing procedure, the next image was obtained **(B)**. Although the pattern of nonuniformity in **A** corresponding to location of PM tubes behind the crystal has been eliminated, some nonuniformity persists (the image in **B** is darker at the lower left than in the center), and further adjustment of the camera was necessary.

the patient, acquiring an image at each of perhaps 60 locations. The resulting multiple images are processed by the computer to reconstruct tomographic slices in the transverse, sagittal, or coronal planes. SPECT imaging improves contrast by reducing the effect of radioactivity in structures outside the slice of interest.

Figure 11–6. Nonuniformity due to cracked crystal. This flood image shows a high degree of uniformity except for the aberration on the right side of the image corresponding to a crack in the crystal.

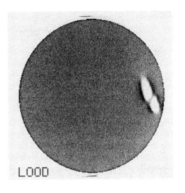

LOOD

Because the distance between the camera and the area of interest is on the average greater than can be obtained with a stationary camera and nontomographic imaging, the spatial resolution of SPECT is poorer than that for nontomographic imaging.

Although camera rotation of 360 degrees around the patient is frequently used, satisfactory images can be reconstructed from partial rotations; 180-degree rotations are often used in cardiac SPECT. Acquisition time can be further reduced if multiple camera heads are used, and cameras are available with two or three heads. An alternative to the rotating camera is a stationary array of collimated detectors that surrounds the patient.

SPECT images are usually acquired in the 64 × 64 or 128 × 128 formats. The minimum slice thickness in the reconstructed tomograms depends on the acquisition format. If desired, adjacent rows of pixel information can be added to improve counting statistics, but this practice results in thicker tomographic slices. Slice thickness is usually adjusted to 15 to 25 mm. Thinner slices are pointless, as the FWHM in most SPECT systems lies between 15 and 20 mm.

Positron Emission Tomography

In the annihilation of a positron and electron, two 511-keV photons are emitted in opposite directions. Two detectors facing each other and oriented along a straight line through the patient can be used to localize these radiation sources along lines through the patient. If the pair of detectors is rotated around the patient, tomographic reconstructions can be done analogous to the method used in SPECT. Alternatively, multiple pairs of stationary detectors can be located around the patient.

The nuclides available for positron emission tomography (PET) imaging are carbon-11, nitrogen-13, oxygen-15, fluorine-18, and bromine-75. These nuclides have short half-lives and are produced in a cyclotron. The requirement of an on-site cyclotron, along with the complexity of the PET camera, make PET installations very expensive. This modality has been used primarily for research, although some clinical installations are in place.

Radiopharmaceutical Chemistry

A radiopharmaceutical is a drug labeled with a radionuclide that, in the case of diagnostic imaging, emits gamma rays or x-rays. The radionuclides of therapeutic radiopharmaceuticals may emit alpha or beta particles, which are useless for imaging but result in high local patient radiation dose.

Tc-99m is the label of most currently used radiopharmaceuticals. This nuclide is eluted from a Mo-99–Tc-99m generator in the form of Tc-99m pertechnetate. Other important radionuclides used for labeling pharmaceuticals are iodine and indium. I-131 is reactor-produced and relatively inexpensive. Its 364-keV gamma radiation is too energetic for ideal imaging, and concomitant beta particles result in high patient radiation dose. I-123 has an ideal 159-keV gamma radiation and a reasonable 13-hour half-life. I-123 is cyclotron produced and thus relatively expensive. In-111 emits 172- and 247-keV gamma particles, emits no beta particles, has a 2.83-day half-life, and is cyclotron produced.

Incorporation of radioiodine into a molecule can be direct or indirect. The commonly used direct techniques are the chloramine-T and iodogen methods. In these methods oxidizing agents convert iodine to the cationic species so that they can replace hydrogen or iodine in the drug molecule. In indirect iodination the iodine is initially bound to a coupling agent that is then coupled to the drug molecule. In-111 is attached to the drug molecule with a chelating agent such as oxine or EDTA.

Many radiopharmaceutical kits are available for the preparation of Tc-99m-labeled radiopharmaceuticals. These kits contain the pharmaceutical in dry form along with a reducing agent such as stannous ion. The reducing agent allows the pertechnetate ion to be complexed to a chelating agent that is also supplied with the kit.

Quality Control

Radiopharmaceutical

Radionuclide purity of Tc-99m is a measure of Mo-99 contaminants. Mo-99 emits 740- and 778-keV gamma photons. Because these photons are much more energetic than the 140-keV gamma photons from Tc-99m, Mo-99 contamination can be estimated by using a special lead shield that stops most 140-keV photons but passes many of the higher-energy Mo-99 photons. Mo-99 radioactivity should be kept below 0.15 µCi/mCi of Tc-99m.

Chemical purity of pertechnetate is a measure of undesirable chemical contamination, usually in the form of aluminum that has been leached from the alumina column of the Tc-99m generator.

Radiochemical purity of Tc-99m is a measure of the percent of the radioactivity contributed by the +7 oxidation state of Tc-99m. Contaminants are Tc-99m in the +4, +5, and +6 oxidation states. These contaminants can be detected with thin-layer chromatography and cause poor labeling of the radiopharmaceutical if present in excessive quantities.

Equipment

The National Electrical Manufacturer's Association (NEMA) has established tests for nuclear medicine imaging systems. These tests are designed to evaluate resolution; uniformity; geometric distortion, including spatial linearity; and system limitations related to both high and low count rates. The calibration of nonimaging instrumentation such as thyroid probes, well counters, and dose calibrators is subject to drift and should also be tested.

Daily testing of the dose calibrator can be done with known standards of cesium-137 and cobalt-57, which have energies of 662 keV, and 122 keV, respectively. These energies simulate those encountered with Mo-99 and Tc-99m. Dose calibrator linearity can be tested by following the decay of a nuclide such as Tc-99m that has a relatively short half-life. Drifting of the electronics and dose calibrators, well counters, and thyroid probes can be followed daily by noting the settings of energy level necessary to obtain maximum response to a known isotope when a narrow window setting is used. This setting may change slightly from day to day, but the change should be minimal and should not show a trend in one direction.

There are no published regulations or guidelines from regulatory agencies concerning quality control equipment testing in nuclear medicine. The guidelines given here are based on published recommendations from academic nuclear medicine sources. Table 11–2 summarizes these guidelines; the table reflects compromises where the published guidelines differ. Gamma cameras used for SPECT imaging may require more frequent attention than is indicated in Table 11–2. In particular, uniformity is a critical parameter that must receive careful attention for successful SPECT imaging. The manufacturer's recommendations concerning uniformity testing and correction should be consulted.

Table 11–2. Summary of Quality Control Testing

	Imaging Equipment	Nonimaging Equipment	Pharmacy
Daily	uniformity; film for matter settings; film processor consistency	dose calibrator accuracy; survey meter accuracy	radiochemical purity
Weekly	spatial resolution; linearity	well counter accuracy	radionuclide purity
Quarterly	energy resolution; collimator integrity	dose calibrator linearity	
Annual	count rate response; multiwindow registration; sensitivity		

Procedures

The procedures described here are intended to be guidelines only. The individual case will frequently require that the procedure be tailored to the specific needs of the case. The doses are appropriate for average-sized adults.

Procedure	Pharmaceutical	Dose	Views	Comments
Bone metabolism	Tc-99m-MDP	25 mCi (925 MBq), i.v.	ANT, POST	500K-count images are acquired 2–3 hr after injection. For 3-phase study, serial 5-sec images are acquired for 1 min following injection; then a 1-min image is acquired.
Brain delayed imaging	Tc-99m-DTPA	25 mCi (925 MBq), i.v.	ANT,LAT, Post, Vertex	This acquisition follows a Tc-99m-DTPA brain perfusion study.
Brain perfusion	I-123-IMP	6 mCi (222 MBq), i.v.	SPECT	Acquisition is started 20 min after injection.
Brain perfusion study	Tc-99m-DTPA	25 mCi (925 MBq), i.v.	ANT	Acquire 2- or 3-sec serial images for 30 sec after injection followed by an immediate 200K-count static image.
Brain perfusion	Tc-99m-HMPAO or Tc99m-ECD	20 mCi (740 MBq), i.v.	SPECT	Acquisition is started 20 min after injection.

Procedure	Pharmaceutical	Dose	Views	Comments
Cisternography	In-111 DTPA intrathecally	1.5 mCi (55.5 MBq)	ANT, LAT, Post	Following lumbar injection 200K-count images are obtained at 2, 6, and 24 hr.
Cystogram	Tc-99m-DTPA	1 mCi	ANT or POST	The Tc-99m-DTPA is administered with saline under low pressure into the bladder. Serial 1-min images are acquired during filling and through voiding.
Gallium imaging	Ga-67 citrate i.v.	6 mCi (222 MBq)	ANT, POST	5–10-min images are acquired at 48 hr or as needed at 6, 24, 48, and 72 hr.
Gastric emptying	Tc-99m-sulfur colloid	1 mCi	ANT	Instant oatmeal is labeled with Tc-99m-sulfur colloid. 1-min images are acquired every 10-15 min following ingestion for 1 hr. Radioactivity is measured in a gastric region of interest.

Procedure	Pharmaceutical	Dose	Views	Comments
Gastroesophageal reflux	Tc-99m-sulfur colloid	300 µCi (11.1 MBq)	ANT	150 mL orange juice and 150 mL 0.1 N HCl are labeled with Tc-99m-sulfur colloid and administered orally. 30-sec images are acquired for sequential pressures of 0–100 mmHg in an abdominal binder. Binder should be used for adults only.
Gastrointestinal bleeding	Tc-99m-RBCs i.v.	25 mCi (925 MBq)	ANT	1-min images are acquired every 1 min for 1 hr, then as necessary up to 36 hr.
Hepatic perfusion and blood pool (for cavernous hemangioma)	Tc-99m-RBCs i.v.	25 mCi (925 MBq)	Perfusion: ANT immediate blood pool: ANT, POST, R LAT, delayed blood pool: SPECT	Perfusion: 3-sec images for 1.5 min. Immediate blood pool: 500K counts; delayed blood pool 60 min after injection: 500K counts.

Procedure	Pharmaceutical	Dose	Views	Comments
Hepatobiliary study	Tc-99m-DISIDA	6 mCi (222 MBq)	ANT, R LAT, RAO	The ANT view is acquired at 5 and 10 min. All views are acquired at 15, 30, 45, and 60, and at delayed times as needed.
Liver–spleen	Tc-99m-sulfur colloid i.v.	6 mCi (222 MBq)	ANT, POST, L LAT, R LAT, RAO, LPO, RPO	A 500K-count ANT image is acquired at 5 min. The other images are acquired for the same time as the ANT image.
Lung perfusion	Tc-99m-MAA i.v.	2–6 mCi	ANT, POST, R LAT, L LAT, LPO, RPO	500K-count images are acquired following injection. 2–3 mCi are used if perfusion imaging is done before ventilation imaging. 4–6 mCi are used if perfusion imaging is done after ventilation imaging

Procedure	Pharmaceutical	Dose	Views	Comments
Lung ventilation	Tc-99m-DTPA aerosol	1–5 mCi	ANT, POST, R LAT, L LAT, LPO, RPO	500K-count images are acquired following inhalation of aerosol. If the ventilation imaging is done before perfusion imaging 1–2 mCi Tc-99m-DTPA aerosol are administered. When ventilation imaging is done after perfusion imaging, administered dose of aerosol should be adjusted so that at least 75% of the total counts in each image are from the Tc-99m-DTPA aerosol.
Lung ventilation	Xe-133	20 mCi (740 MBq)	POST	An image is acquired during breath holding after inhalation of a single deep breath of Xe-

Procedure	Pharmaceutical	Dose	Views	Comments
				133. The acquisition time is as long as the patient can suspend respiration. Then the patient breathes Xe-133 plus air normally for 3 min or until the monitor shows stabilization of the distribution of Xe-133 in the lungs; a 300K-count image is acquired. Then the patient breathes into an exhaust system, and serial 30-sec images are acquired for 2 min or until the monitor shows absent residual Xe-133 in the lungs.
Lymphoscintigraphy	Tc-99m-HSA or: Tc99m antimony trisulfide colloid if available or; filtered Tc99m sulfur colloid (0.1-0.2 micron)	Up to 7mCi intradermally	ANT	Acquire images at 1, 5, 15, 30, 45, and 60 min. Later images as necessary for evaluation of lymphedema.

Procedure	Pharmaceutical	Dose	Views	Comments
Marrow imaging	Tc-99m-sulfur colloid i.v.	15 mCi (555 MBq)	ANT, POST	2-min images are acquired of the body regions of interest beginning 15 min after injection.
Meckel's diverticulum	Tc-99m-pertechnetate	5 mCi, i.v.	ANT	500K-count images are acquired at 1, 5, 10, 15, 30, 45, and 60 min after injection. Susequent images every 15 min may be indicated.
MUGA	Tc-99m-RBCs	25 mCi, i.v.	ANT, LAO (L LAT, RAO)	Serial 1-sec images can be done for first pass. Exercise MUGA requires serial 2.5-min acquisitions at increasing exercise levels followed by a 2.5 min postexercise acquisition.
Myocardial infarct	Tc-99m-pyrophosphate	25 mCi, i.v.	RAO, ANT LAO, L LAT	3 hr, 500K-counts each.

Procedure	Pharmaceutical	Dose	Views	Comments
Myocardial perfusion	Tc-99m-sestamibi, i.v. Tc-99m-tetrofosmin, i.v.	(see right)	SPECT	rest: 10-mCi; acquisition started 15 min after injection. Stress: 25 mCi injection 1 to 2 min before end of exercise. Acquisition started 15 min after injection.
Myocardial perfusion	Tc-99m-teboroxime i.v.	25 (925 MBq) mCi, i.v.	SPECT	Pharmaceutical injection during exercise followed by a 10 min data acquisition. A second injection and data acquisition are done 1 hr later.
Myocardial perfusion	Thallium-201	2–3 mCi (111 MBq) at stress, 10 min prior to imaging	SPECT	For stress, injection 1-2 min before termination of exercise.
		1–2 mCi (74 MBq) 5 min prior to rest imaging	SPECT	For rest, reinjection may also be done after stress image acquisition completed, followed by 2-3 hour delay.

263

Procedure	Pharmaceutical	Dose	Views	Comments
Parathyroid imaging	Tl-201 and Tc-99m-pertechnetate or: Tc99m-sestamibi 25 mCi, i.v.	3 mCi (111 MBq), i.v. 10 mCi (370 MBq), i.v.	ANT	The Tl-201 acquisition is done first, 30 min after injection. The Tc-99m-pertechnetate acquisition is then done 20 min after injection.100K-count images are acquired.
Pulmonary aspiration	Tc-99m-sulfur colloid	2 mCi, oral	ANT, POST	The patient is instructed to retire immediately after ingesting tracer in 300mL water. 5-min images are acquired the next morning.
Renal imaging, glomerular filtration	Tc-99m-DTPA	15 mCi (555 MBq), i.v.	POST (ANT for transplants)	Serial 2- or 3-sec images are obtained for 1-min, followed by serial 1- or 2-min images for 20 min.
Renal Cortical Imaging, Differential Function	Tc-99m-DMSA i.v.	5 mCi (185 MBq)	POST, LPO, RPO	500K-count images are acquired 3 hr after injection.

Procedure	Pharmaceutical	Dose	Views	Comments
Renal Imaging, Tubular secretion	Tc-99m-MAG3 i.v.	10 mCi (370 MBq)	Same as for Tc-99m-DTPA	Imaging is same as for Tc-99m-DTPA.
Renal Imaging, Tubular secretion	I-131 Hippuran i.v.	350 μCi (13 MBq)	Same as for Tc-99m-DTPA	Serial 3-min images are acquired for 24 min; no flow study.
Testicular perfusion	Tc-99m-pertechnetate	15 mCi (555 MBq)	ANT	Serial 5-sec images are acquired for 45 sec, followed by 750K-count static images at 1, 5, and 10 min.
Thyroid uptake	I-123 or I-131	0.5 mCi (18.5 MBq) oral 10 μCi (0.37MBq) oral		The dose activity in a neck phantom is first measured with a probe. The probe is then used to measure neck activity in the patient 4 hr and 24 hr after administration. The uptake is expressed as a percentage of the phantom radioactivity and is corrected for background and decay.

Thyroid imaging	I-123	0.5 mCi (18.5 MBq), oral	ANT, both anterior obliques	100K-count images are acquired 24 hrs after I-123 administration. Alternative is to acquire at 6 hrs.
Thyroid imaging	Tc-99m-pertechnetate i.v.	5 mCi (185 MBq)	ANT, both anterior obliques	Acquisition is done 20 min after administration of Tc-99m-pertechnetate. 200K-count images are acquired.
Whole-body I-131 imaging (metastatic survey)	II-131 orally	5-10 mCi (185-370 MBq)	ANT, POST	5-min images are acquired 48 to 72 hr after administration.
White blood cell imaging	In-111-oxine WBCs	0.5 mCi, i.v.	ANT, POST	5–10-min images are acquired at 4 or 6 hrs and at 24 hr and as needed at 48 hr.
	or: Tc99m-HMPAO WBC's	10mCi (370 MBq), i.v.	ANT, POST	Acquisition begins at 2 hrs.

Radiopharmaceuticals Used in Scintigraphy

Pharmaceutical	Organ	rad/mCi = mGy/3.7 MBq
Ga-67 citrate	Colon	0.90
	Testes	0.24
	Whole body	0.26
	Ovaries	0.28
	Small intestine	0.36
	Kidneys	0.41
	Liver	0.46
	Spleen	0.53
	Marrow	0.58
In-111-DTPA	Whole body	0.082
(2-hr void)	Testes	0.08
	Ovaries	0.12
	Bladder	0.42
	Kidneys	0.44
	Brain (surface)	8.1
	Spinal cord (surface)	10.0
In-111-MAb B72.3	Testes	0.24
	Thyroid	0.30
	Whole body	0.54
	Uterus	0.54
	Bladder	0.56
	Ovaries	0.58
	Small intestine	0.60
	Colon	0.62
	Heart	0.64
	Stomach	0.64
	Bone	0.66
	Pancreas	0.74
	Adrenals	0.90
	Lungs	0.98
	Kidneys	1.94
	Marrow	2.4
	Liver	3.0
	Spleen	3.2

Pharmaceutical	Organ	rad/mCi = mGy/3.7 MBq
In-111-WBCs (assumes 0.25% In-114m)	Testes	0.028
	Ovaries	0.40
	Whole body	0.74
	Marrow	4.0
	Liver	5.4
	Spleen	40.0
I-123 (for 15% maximum thyroid uptake)	Liver	0.038
	Whole body	0.043
	Testes	0.048
	Marrow	0.04
	Ovaries	0.08
	Stomach	0.24
	Thyroid	7.3
I-131(for 15% maximum thyroid uptake)	Testes	0.85
	Marrow	0.20
	Ovaries	0.14
	Liver	0.35
	Whole body	0.47
	Stomach	1.6
	Thyroid	800.00
I-131-Hippuran	Kidneys	0.08
	Testes	0.11
	Whole body	0.11
	Ovaries	0.13
	Bladder	5.7
Tc-99m-DMSA	Testes	0.007
	Ovaries	0.013
	Whole body	0.015
	Marrow	0.022
	Liver	0.032
	Bladder	0.07
	Kidneys	0.85
Tc-99m-DTPA (2-hr void) (intravenous)	Whole body	0.006
	Testes	0.008
	Ovaries	0.01
	Kidneys	0.09
	Bladder	0.12
Tc-99m-DTPA (instilled into bladder)	Ovaries	0.002
	Bladder	0.025

Pharmaceutical	Organ	rad/mCi = mGy/3.7 MBq
Tc-99m-DTPA Aerosol	Kidneys	0.02
	Whole body	0.02
	Lungs	0.05
	Bladder	0.1
Tc-99m-glucoheptonate (2-hr void)	Testes	0.008
	Liver	0.012
	Ovaries	0.013
	Bladder	0.12
	Kidneys	0.24
Tc-99m-HMPAO	Testes	0.007
	Whole body	0.013
	Ovaries	0.024
	Brain	0.025
	Small intestine	0.044
	Liver	0.054
	Colon	0.079
	Thyroid	0.10
	Kidneys	0.13
	Gallbladder	0.19
	Lacrimal	0.26
Tc-99m-human serum albumin (intravenous)	Brain	0.009
	Kidneys	0.011
	Total body	0.015
	Marrow	0.015
	Testes	0.016
	Ovaries	0.016
	Bladder	0.033
Tc-99m-MAA (2-hr void)	Testes	0.006
	Ovaries	0.008
	Kidneys	0.011
	Whole body	0.015
	Spleen	0.017
	Liver	0.018
	Bladder wall	0.03
	Lungs	0.22
Tc-99m-MAG3	Liver	0.004
	Marrow	0.005
	Whole body	0.007
	Kidneys	0.014

Pharmaceutical	Organ	rad/mCi = mGy/3.7 MBq
	Testes	0.016
	Ovaries	0.026
	Colon	0.033
	Bladder	0.48
Tc-99m-MDP (2-hr void	Whole body	0.0065
	Liver	0.003
	Testes	0.008
	Ovaries	0.012
	Marrow	0.028
	Bone	0.035
	Kidneys	0.04
	Bladder	0.13
Tc-99m-mebrofenin	Testes	0.005
	Marrow	0.034
	Liver	0.047
	Whole body	0.02
	Bladder	0.03
	Ovaries	0.10
	Gallbladder	0.14
	Small intestine	0.29
	Colon	0.47
Tc-99m-octreotide	Testes	0.10
	Ovaries	0.16
	Adrenals	0.25
	Thyroid	0.25
	Colon	0.26
	Liver	0.41
	Whole body	0.43
	Bladder	1.0
	Kidneys	1.81
	Spleen	2.46
Tc-99m-pertechnetate (intravenous; active population)	Testes	0.009
	Whole body	0.011
	Marrow	0.017
	Stomach	0.051
	Bladder	0.085
	Ovaries	0.03
	Colon	0.12
	Thyroid	0.13

Pharmaceutical	Organ	rad/mCi = mGy/3.7 MBq
Tc-99m-pertechnetate (ocular)	Testes	0.009
	Total body	0.011
	Ovaries	0.030
	Thyroid	0.13
	Lens	0.22 (no blockage
		4.0 (complete blockage
Tc-99m-pyrophosphate (2-hr void)	Total body	0.015
	Marrow	0.038
	Kidneys	0.047
	Bone	0.054
	Ovaries	0.01
	Testes	0.01
	Bladder	0.10
Tc-99m-RBCs	Testes	0.011
	Marrow	0.015
	Whole body	0.015
	Ovaries	0.016
	Bone	0.024
	Liver	0.029
	Blood	0.04
	Heart	0.10
	Spleen	0.11
	Kidneys	0.23
Tc-99m-sestamibi (2-hr void)	Testes	0.010
	Marrow	0.017
	Whole body	0.017
	Thyroid	0.023
	Ovaries	0.050
	Bladder	0.067
	Gallbladder	0.067
	Kidneys	0.067
	Liver	0.02
	Small bowel	0.10
	Colon	0.18
Tc-99m-sulfur colloid (intravenous)	Testes	0.0011
	Ovaries	0.006
	Whole body	0.019
	Marrow	0.028

Pharmaceutical	Organ	rad/mCi = mGy/3.7 MBq
	Spleen	0.21
	Liver	0.34
Tc-99m-sulfur colloid (oral)	Testes	0.004
	Whole body	0.018
	Ovaries	0.08
	Stomach	0.14
	Small intestine	0.26
	Colon	0.48
Tc-99m-teboroxime	Testes	0.010
	Marrow	0.017
	Whole body	0.017
	Kidneys	0.020
	Heart	0.020
	Bladder	0.027
	Lungs	0.028
	Ovaries	0.036
	Liver	0.062
	Small intestine	0.068
	Gallbladder	0.10
	Colon	0.12
T1-201	Whole body	0.21
	Colon	0.25
	Small intestine	0.38
	Stomach	0.42
	Ovaries	0.47
	Heart	0.50
	Testes	0.50
	Liver	0.55
	Thyroid	0.65
	Kidneys	1.20
Xe-133	Brain	0.00005
	Whole body	0.00009
	Lungs	0.0083

References to Appendix II

Mediphysics DTPA package insert. 1985.
Mediphysics Tc-99m-MAA package insert. 1984.
Squibb Diagnostic Tc-99m-Choletec package insert. 1992.
DuPont Merck Tc-99m-Pyrolite package insert. 1991.

Amersham Tc-99m-DMSA package insert. 1993.
New England Tc-99m-Glucoscan package insert. 1991.
Mediphysics Tc-99m-HSA package insert. 1984.
Amersham Tc-99m-MDP package insert. 1987.
Mediphysics Tc-99m-TSC package insert. 1988.
Mallinckrodt In-111-Octreoscan package insert. 1994.
Mallinckrodt UltraTag Tc-99m-RBC kit package insert. 1992.
Mallinckrodt Tednescan MAG3 kit package insert. 1992.
DuPont Merck Tc-99m-Cardiolite list package insert. 1992.
Sqibb Tc-99m-Cardiolite package insert. 1992.
Amersham Tc-99m-Ceretec package insert. 1995.
DuPont Gallium Citrate package insert. 1993.
Amersham In-111-Oxyquimoline package insert. 1994.
Mediphysics MPI Indium package insert. 1990.
Cytogen In-111-Oncoscint package insert. 1992.
Mediphysics I-123 package insert. 1992.
CIS bio I-131 package insert. 1990.
Mallinckrodt I-131-Hippuran package insert. 1992.
DuPont Merck T1-201-Chloride package insert. 1991.
DuPont Merck Xe-133 Gas package insert. 1994.
DuPont Merck Technelite Tc-99m generator package insert. 1993.

Isotopes Used in Scintigraphy

Isotope	Radiation type	Mean % per disintegration	Half-life	Mean Energy (keV)
Ga-67			3.26 days	
	Gamma-2	38.3		93.3
	Gamma-3	20.9		184.6
	Gamma-5	16.8		300.2
	Gamma-6	4.7		393.5
In-111			2.83 days	
	Gamma-2	90.2		171.0
	Gamma-3	94.0		245.0
I-123	Gamma-2	83.3	13.2 hr	159.0
	Ce-K, gamma-2	13.6		127.0
I-131			8.04 days	
	Beta-4	89.4		191.0
	Gamma-14	81.2		364.0
Tc-99m	Gamma-2	89.0	6hr	140.5
T1-201	Gamma-4	2.7	3.05 days	135.3
	Gamma-6	10.0		167.4
	Ce-K, gamma-8	15.4		84.3
	K alpha-1 x-ray	46.2		70.8
	K alpha-2 x-ray	27.2		68.9
	K beta-1 x-ray	10.5		80.3
Xe-133			5.25 days	
	Beta-2	99.3		100.5
	Ce-K-2	52.0		45.0
	Ce-L-2	8.5		75.3
	Ce-M-2	2.3		79.8
	Gamma-2	37.1		81.0
	K alpha-2 x-ray	13.3		30.6
	K alpha-1 x-ray	24.6		31.0
	K beta x-rays	8.8		35.0
P-32	Beta		14.3 days	695.0
Sr-89	Beta		50.5 days	583.0

Rules and Regulations

This summary is taken from the Nuclear Regulatory Commission's rules and regulations that apply to the medical use of radioisotopes, and is intended to be a guide rather than an exhaustive review. Further detail can be obtained from the code of Federal Regulations Title 10, Chapter 1, Parts 19, 20, 30, and 35.

License

The NRC requires that anyone who manufactures, acquires, possesses, or uses medical radioisotopes do so under an appropriate license. When the user is part of a medical institution, the institution's management must apply for the license. If the user is not part of a medical institution, then this individual must apply.

ALARA Program

The licensee must develop a radiation protection program in which radiation doses are kept as low as reasonably achievable (ALARA). All users must participate in this program. The program must include a review of summaries of the types and amounts of radioisotopes used along with radioactive doses to personnel. Continuing education and training must be provided for all personnel who work with or near the radioisotopes.

Radiation Safety Officer

A radiation safety officer (RSO), responsible for implementing a radiation safety program, must be appointed by the licensee. The RSO investigates deviations from approved practice. These deviations include over exposures, accidents, spills, losses, and unauthorized use of radioisotopes. The RSO develops policies and procedures for purchasing, receiving, and storing radioisotopes and keeps an inventory of the radioisotopes. The written policy should also specify the safe use of isotopes and the emergency action necessary in accidents, periodic radiation surveys and the periodic testing of survey instruments, how isotopes are disposed of, how personnel will be trained in the use of isotopes, and the means of record keeping.

The RSO is required to brief the institution's management on the program. The RSO establishes personnel radiation exposure levels at which the RSO will investigate the exposure.

Radiation Safety Committee

The NRC requires that each institution have a radiation safety committee to oversee the use of radioisotopes. This committee must consist of at least three individuals including the RSO. The committee meets at least quarterly and discusses the ALARA program, the qualifications of potential users of radionuclides, changes in radiation safety procedures, personnel dose records, and accidents. The committee should review the radiation safety program annually.

Quality Management Program

Each licensee must have a quality management program, the purpose of which is to ensure that the radionuclides will be administered as directed by the authorized user. This program requires written orders for radionuclide therapy or for the administration of greater than 30 µCi of I-125 or I-131. Accidental deviations from the written orders must be evaluated and appropriate action taken. Within 30 days of any deviation from the written order, the licensee must inform the NRC of the event and provide a proposal for a change in the quality management program to increase the program's efficiency.

Misadministrations

Following a misadministration, the licensee must notify the NRC no later than the following calendar day after the discovery of the misadministration. Within 15 days of the misadministration, a written report must be submitted that includes a description of the event and what measures will be taken to prevent future occurrences. The referring physician must also be notified no longer than 24 hours after the discovery of a misadministration. Either the referring physician or the licensee should inform the patient within 24 hours unless the referring physician deems that this would be harmful to the patient.

Suppliers

Therapeutic and diagnostic radiopharmaceuticals must be manufactured, labeled, packaged, and distributed according to NRC regulations.

Technical Requirements

The licensee must have a dose calibrator to measure the amount of radioactivity that each patient receives. This device must be tested for constancy daily, for accuracy at least annually, for linearity at least quarterly, and for geometry dependance at the time of installation.

Radiation survey instruments must be calibrated annually and should be accurate to within 20%. If the indicated exposure rate differs from the calculated exposure rate by more than 20%, then a correction chart can be used.

Radiopharmaceutical doses over 10 µCi must be measured before use. Doses below 10 µCi must be measured to ascetain that they are below this level. Records of these measurements must be kept for 3 years.

Sealed sources must be tested for leakage every 6 months. This test is accomplished by a wipe of the source or its container. If the radioactivity on the wipe sample is greater than .005 µCi the source must be placed in storage, and the NRC informed of the leak. Records of leakage testing must be kept for 3 years.

Syringes used for radiopharmaceutical administration must be kept in a radiation shield; the syringe must be labeled with the radiopharmaceutical and the patient's name. Those who prepare radiopharmaceuticals must use a syringe radiation shield during the preparation and a syringe shield when administering the pharmaceutical.

A survey instrument must be used at the end of each day to check all areas of radiopharmaceutical preparation for contamination. Areas where radiopharmaceuticals or waste are stored must be checked weekly. The licensee must establish radiation trigger levels above which the RSO will be informed. Wipe tests must be done weekly on areas in which radiopharmaceuticals are routinely prepared, administered, or stored, and trigger levels should be established above which the radiation safety officer will be notified. Records of these surveys must be kept for 3 years.

Patients having radiopharmaceuticals or radioactive implants may not be released from the hospital until either the measured dose rate from the patient is less than 5mR/hr at a distance of 1 m or until the patient's radioactivity is less than 30 μCi.

The NRC requires that mobile nuclear medicine services transport only syringes or vials containing prepared pharmaceuticals or radiopharmaceuticals intended for reconstitutions from kits. Surveys for contamination must be carried out at the client's address before the mobile unit leaves the address after each use.

Disposal of Medical Radioisotopes

Isotopes with half lives less than 65 days may be disposed of in ordinary trash after they have been held for decay for at least 10 half lives. The material being disposed of must be surveyed to confirm that the radioactivity level from the material cannot be ditinguished from the background radiation level. Records of such disposal must be kept for 3 years.

Use of Diagnostic Radiopharmaceuticals

Radiopharmaceuticals used diagnostically must be approved by the Food and Drug Administration (FDA) either through acceptance of an investigational new drug exemption application (IND) or an approved new drug application (NDA). Molybdenum-99 contamination of Tc-99m obtained from a generator must not exceed 0.15 μCi of molybdenum-99 per millicurie of Tc-99m. The contamination level must be measured in each eluate from the generator. Records of these measurements must be kept for 3 years.

Radioactive gases used diagnostically must be administered in rooms that are kept at negative pressure relative to surrounding rooms. The administration system must either vent the gas to the atmosphere through an exhaust system or provide for collection and decay in a shielded container.

Therapeutic Radiopharmaceuticals

Therapeutic radiopharmaceuticals must be accepted by the FDA either through an IND or an NDA. Instruction must be provided to all personnel caring for patients receiving radiopharmaceutical therapy. Each patient must be provided a private room with a private bathroom. The room's door should be posted with a sign reading "radioactive material". On the door or on the patients records should be a note indicating where and how long visitors may stay in the patient's room. Visitors under 18 must be admitted only with the approval of the RSO. Shortly after the administration of the therapeutic dose, surrounding rooms should be surveyed. Objects taken from the patient's room can be released only when their radioactivity cannot be distinguished from background. The patient's room must be surveyed and found to have wipe test contamination less than 200 disintegrations per minute per 100 square centimeters before another person is assigned to the room. Personnel who help prepare or administer therapeutic I-131 should be measured for thyroid burden within three days of the administration. The RSO must be notified immediately if a patient dies or has a medical emergency.

Training Requirements

Physicians authorized to use radiopharmaceuticals diagnostically for uptake, dilution, and excretion studies must be certified in nuclear medicine by the American Board of Nuclear Medicine or diagnostic radiology by the American Board of Radiology or diagnostic radiology or radiology by the American Osteopathic Board of Radiology. Physicians can use radiopharmaceuticals diagnostically without the above board requirements if they have 40 hours of classroom and laboratory training including radiation physics, radiation protection, mathematics pertaining to radioactivity, radiation biology, and radiopharmaceutical chemistry, and 20 hours of clinical experience supervised by an authorized user; in addition, these users must complete a 6-month training program in nuclear medicine approved by the accreditation council for graduate medical education. The requirements for a user performing imaging and localization studies rather than just uptake dilution and excretion studies are similar except that 200 hours of classroom and laboratory training and 500 hours of supervised experience are required.

Users performing therapy with radiopharmaceuticals must be certified by the American Board of Nuclear Medicine or the American Board of Radiology or have 80 hours of classroom and laboratory training. They must have had supervised experience using I-131 to treat 10 patients with hyperthyroidism and 3 patients with thyroid carcinoma.

Occupational Exposure Dose Limits

Table A.IV-1 summarizes the NRC occupational dose limits. Occupational exposures to minors are limited to 10% of those shown in the table. The dose to an embryo or a fetus may not exceed .005 Sv (0.5 rem); this regulation applies to women who have voluntarily declared themselves to be pregnant. The dose limit to individuals in the public should not exceed 1mSv (100 mrems) per year.

Table AIV-1. NRC Radiation Dose Limits

Region	Occupational Radiation Dose Limit
Lens	150 mSv(15 rem)/yr
Skin, hands, feet	500 mSv(50 rem)/yr
Any tissue	500 mSv(50 rem)/yr
Embryo or fetus	5 mSv(0.5 rem)/duration of pregnancy
Total effective dose	50 mSv(5 rem)/yr

Index

Page numbers in *italics* refer to illustrations; page numbers followed by t indicate tables.

282